Organizing AIDS

Social Aspects of AIDS
Series Editor: Peter Aggleton
Institute of Education, University of London

Organizing AIDS:
Workplace and Organizational Responses to the HIV/AIDS Epidemic

David Goss and Derek Adam-Smith

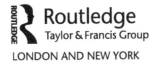

Routledge
Taylor & Francis Group

LONDON AND NEW YORK

First published 1995 by Taylor & Francis

Published 2021 by Routledge
2 Park Square, Milton Park, Abingdon, Oxon OX14 4RN
605 Third Avenue, New York, NY 10017

Routledge is an imprint of the Taylor & Francis Group, an informa business

ISBN 13: 978-0-7484-0258-8 (hbk)
ISBN 13: 978-0-7484-0259-5 (pbk)

A Catalogue Record for this book is available from the British Library

**Library of Congress Cataloging-in-Publication Data are available on
request**

Typeset in 11/13 pt Baskerville
by Solidus (Bristol) Limited

Contents

Acknowledgments

We are indebted to a number of people and organizations without whose help and cooperation the completion of this book would not have been possible. The fieldwork research reported in the book was supported by the Economic and Social Research Council (grant number R000 234131) and we record our gratitude to those organizations, managers and staff who gave freely of their time to answer our questions. Thanks also to three of our colleagues at Portsmouth: Karen Meudell and Karen Gadd who undertook a number of the interviews, and Adele Sinclair who commented on earlier drafts of Chapters six and seven. We are also grateful for the support given to us by Vanessa Hardy and her colleagues at the National AIDS Trust. Finally, special thanks to Fiona, Sophie, Charlotte, Dilys and Kip for their patience and good humour while we spent too many unsocial hours at the word processor.

David Goss and Derek Adam-Smith, January 1995

Series Editor's Preface

Since the earliest days of the epidemic, people with HIV and AIDS, and people presumed to be infected, have been subjected to discrimination, ostracization and even dismissal from their place of employment. Efforts have often been made to justify such actions on public health grounds or in terms of responsiveness to the anxieties and demands of co-workers. But as David Goss and Derek Adam-Smith show, these responses conceal a more hidden agenda linked to enduring anxieties about 'normality' and 'abnormality', and social as well as virological contagion. Of course, there have also been attempts to foster more supportive workplace and organizational responses towards people living with HIV, spearheaded by affected communities, enlightened public health workers and community organizations working for those affected. While not uncontested, such actions have contributed towards a more realistic appreciation of HIV disease and its work-related consequences. This book charts the origins, emergence and effects of both of the above dominant patterns of response. It does so with a view to offering employers, managers, researchers and organizational theorists insight into some of the more productive ways in which HIV can be tackled in the workplace. Using case study material from a range of countries, and in an engaging and accessible manner, the authors point to ways in which anxieties and fears can be successfully challenged through good workplace policy and practice.

Peter Aggleton

Chapter 1

AIDS, Employment and the Workplace

Introduction

This book is about the various ways in which people have responded to the HIV/AIDS epidemic in their roles as employers, employees, and the users of services provided by employing organizations. This is an area that has been largely ignored by researchers investigating the social implications of AIDS, a neglect that probably stems from a number of inter-related factors. Firstly, the workplace is not generally associated with behaviours which lead to the transmission of HIV, i.e., the 'recreational' activities of sex and drug-use. Secondly, for many of those who have become ill as a result of HIV infection, work is not an option. Indeed, many are encouraged by advisers to give up work at an early opportunity in order to gain full access to state benefits or to avoid stress or exertion that could further impair their health (Green, 1995). Finally, there is the view, particularly common in western Europe with its well developed culture of state welfare provision, that issues relating to HIV/AIDS, whether they be concerned with prevention, treatment or care, are principally the responsibility of 'expert' state agencies or voluntary/community organizations, rather than the employer. Without necessarily denying some validity to these propositions, it can also be argued that there are important reasons why the sphere of employment and work-related activity should be a focus for HIV/AIDS research.

Actual and Perceived Risk of Transmission

Virtually all guidance and opinion makes clear that there is virtually no risk of transmitting HIV through normal workplace activity. Even in the field of medicine where there is a very small chance of transmission (usually from patient to medical worker rather than vice versa) this can be drastically reduced if standard procedures and precautions are followed (Shanson and Cockcroft, 1991). However, a low level of objective risk is not necessarily perceived or accepted as such, and the fear of contracting the virus from some forms of work-related activity has by no means disappeared. Scepticism and uncertainty about possible transmission routes of the virus are prevalent (see, chapter 5 below) and employees infected with HIV, especially if they are employed in caring professions, continue to be the focus of media sensationalism, often with severe ramifications for those directly and indirectly affected. In a very recent case, for example, newspapers initially named the wrong doctor, before 'forcing' the publication of the infected doctor's identity. The UK Sunday newspaper *The People*, for instance, has also focused on a HIV positive doctor and dentist (characterized throughout as 'perverts' [*sic*]) to promote calls for the universal and regular testing of all medical workers to 'protect us' (*The People*, 15 January, 1995). Perceptions of risk inform action and attitudes regardless of the accuracy or otherwise of the information upon which they are based and, as such, may have important implications for the treatment of clients or colleagues thought to be infected.

Although the risk of HIV infection through 'normal' work activity is, indeed, negligible — either because no risk exists or, as in medical work, because potential risks are controlled by specific procedures — there is one area of work where a real prospect of infection may be present, namely, sex work (see, chapter 5 below). Prostitution in particular, may put both women and men at risk as the result either of engaging in unprotected sex (through necessity, coercion or ignorance, see Morgan Thomas, 1992; Maciver, 1992) or from involvement in the practices of drug use that are associated with some areas of this trade (Plant, 1990).

Similarly, there is evidence to suggest that certain indirectly work-related activities may expose people to risk of infection. This applies particularly to workers who spend long periods travelling or working away from home (e.g., seafarers, lorry drivers) who may make greater use of male and female prostitutes or those, such as hospitality industry workers, whose work facilitates opportunities for casual sexual encounters with, for example, visiting tourists. Bloor (1995), for instance, reports a study of 386 migrant tourist industry workers in the UK resort of Torbay, only seven per cent of whom had not engaged in intercourse in the past year, with nearly half of the male workers reporting intercourse with four or more tourists. Overall, only 40 per cent reported condom use during their last intercourse, with use being lowest among those with the most partners.

The Workplace as an Arena of Discrimination and Prejudice

The most widely discussed issue of relevance within the workplace has been that of prejudice and discrimination against people with HIV/ AIDS, be they employees or customers/clients of an organization (see, for example, Wilson, 1995; Panos, 1990; Watt, 1992). This is an issue that has attracted comment around issues of legality, social justice, education and business ethics both in the USA and Europe (Goss, 1993; Patton, 1990; Vest *et al*, 1991). However, in addition to action directed against people with HIV/AIDS as such, the arrival of the epidemic has also exposed more clearly pre-existing tensions and conflicts around issues of sexuality, race, and disability. The emergence of the epidemic has thus fuelled homophobia and racism such that discrimination against homosexuals (including lesbians, stigmatized 'by association' (Richardson, 1994)) and those with presumed African connections can be heightened by being cast in the role of 'viral vector' (Wilson, 1994). This is exemplified by the reporting of a recent UK 'health scandal' in *The People* tabloid newspaper: 'The perverted double life that a dead AIDS dentist and a doctor now dying of the disease ... Inside the perverted world of two MEN who got AIDS and betrayed their patients ... But behind the curtain of respectability lay a sleazy world involving a conveyor belt of gay sex partners' (*The People*, 15 January 1995). Thus, what is clear from services providing advice and guidance to people with HIV/AIDS, is that despite a relatively low number of cases decided before an industrial tribunal (see, chapter six below), discrimination, prejudice and harassment within the work-place, often resulting in the loss of a job, either through dismissal or forced resignation, are by no means uncommon.

The Workplace as an Arena for Support and Assistance

However, against the evidence of discrimination there is also the need to recognize that some employing organizations have been in the forefront of countering prejudice and providing practical assistance to people affected by the virus, both through constructive policies and procedures and support for health education aimed at preventing further infection. In the USA, for instance, considerable attention has been given to the activities of Levi Strauss in its open support for employees with HIV/AIDS, its contribution to AIDS-support organizations, and its opposition to repressive legislation targeted at homosexuals and people with HIV/AIDS (Kohl *et al*, 1990; see, also Kirp, 1989). In the UK, the Body Shop has been regarded as a pioneer in progressive workplace education about HIV/AIDS and both the National AIDS Trust and the Terrence Higgins Trust have found considerable levels of support from major corporate organizations in developing workplace education and support programmes (Belgrave, 1995; IDS, 1993a).

It is also widely accepted that employment provides an important component of identity and a source of psychological support for many people, over and above the material benefits that it brings. Although such attachments may be undermined by expressions of prejudice and discrimination, for many people with HIV work is likely to remain an important component of their lives.

Work as Financial Necessity

The availability of employment for people with HIV infection, however, is also likely to become increasingly significant as changes in the funding and support for health care become increasingly stretched, either as the result of a growing number of people ill with AIDS, as in many developing nations (Merson, 1995), or as the result of cuts in funding in some industrialized countries as the epidemic loses its political impact (Francis, 1993). Already this is an issue in the USA, where contributions to health insurance through employment can have a crucial impact upon the nature and extent of care provided in the event of incapacity. As European governments appear to be placing a greater emphasis on individual contributions to health care funding, such concerns are likely to spread, often meaning that people may need to remain in work for longer, perhaps at the expense of their long-term well-being (see, chapter 4 below) to ensure their health needs are met (Cameron, 1993, p. 101f).

The Epidemic and Those Affected

The demographic profile of the epidemic has focused attention upon the micro and macro-level consequences of infection for employment. Because most of those infected with HIV are in the age groups that have the highest level of economic activity — around half of all known infections are in those between the ages of 15 and 24 (Merson, 1995) — the potential impact on various aspects of employment has always been an issue of concern to governments and employers. This concern was heightened in the western economies during the later 1980s by the fear of massive heterosexual infection coupled with expectations of continuing high levels of economic growth and consequent skill shortages.

In the US where the potential impact of AIDS on employee medical insurance was immediately apparent, concern was widely voiced in the business press. Hamilton (1987) for instance, estimated productivity lost through illness and death associated with AIDS at $55bn and Sullivan (1991) put the cost of AIDS in terms of health and life insurance estimated at $1bn in 1989, a cumulative $2.38bn since 1986. This has been put in stark, if somewhat sensationalist terms, as part of the rationale for a recent European conference aimed at employers:

> $50 billion is the estimated cost of lost productivity, lost markets and retraining incurred last year by the world economy. HIV and AIDS predominantly affects the economically most impor-tant age group, 25–40 year olds — in the UK 90 per cent of HIV positive men are between 20 and 49 years of age — the prime period when your managers, skilled workforce and most highly motivated staff yield their greatest return on your investment — and women are equally AT RISK.
> (capitalization in original) [promotional material, undated]

In the western economies, however, the apparent slowing of the spread of the virus has limited the impact upon aggregate employment levels, making it an issue that is more likely to be experienced at the level of the isolated organization rather than the economy as a whole. Simultaneously, improvements in the medical treatment of AIDS-related illnesses and better understanding of health maintenance during the period of asymptomatic infection also means that, in the western industrial nations, more people are living healthily for longer with the virus and being able to remain relatively fit between bouts of illness at later stages in the syndrome. In this respect, the widely held view of HIV infection as an immediate death sentence is no longer valid, and further points to the viability of keeping those who wish it in employment.

However, it is in Africa and Asia that the greatest impact on employment in more general terms is occurring. In Uganda, for instance, the cost of AIDS is reckoned at 12 per cent of Gross Domestic Product (GDP), coupled to declines in the productivity of subsistence agriculture resulting from the severe decline in the number of working adults. The Uganda Railway Corporation, one of the country's largest employers has lost some 10 per cent of its workforce to AIDS, has seen a tripling of its medical costs, and a massive escalation in days lost through illness (Bellos, 1994, p. 20). A similar picture is painted of Zambia (Merson, 1995, op cit) and Zimbabwe (Jackson and Pitts, 1991).

Having identified ways in which employment and the workplace can influence, and be influenced by, the experience — both individual and collective — of the epidemic, the following sections sketch out some of the more specific factors that have shaped these influences and their effects.

Historical Development of the Epidemic and Organizational Responses

It is now widely recognized that the understanding of AIDS and the social responses to it have passed through a number of stages, informed by a range of discourses from the medical to the moral, and the political to the pragmatic. Thus, according to Berridge (1992) responses to AIDS throughout western societies have followed a broadly three stage pattern. The initial stage (from 1981 to 1986) was that of policy development from below, characterized by relatively limited government/official action, but considerable effort on the part of groups directly affected (Altman, 1994). In this period there was little scientific agreement about the virus, growing media attention and the emergence of public concern and anxiety, leading to the stigmatization and identification of putative 'risk-groups'.

This was followed in 1986–7 by a 'quasi wartime emergency' in which government bodies entered the debate and sought to establish strategic policy and funding initiatives in terms of medical research and social welfare activity, especially health education (see, also, Schramm-Evans, 1990).

Since 1988 there has developed a period of 'normalization' of AIDS facilitated by an apparent slowing of the spread of the virus in western societies (at least when compared with many of the cataclysmic predications of earlier years) with a consequent loss of public and media interest, and a decline in the near-panic engendered during what has been termed the previous 'grim reaper' phases (Lupton, 1994a).

There is certainly an identifiable level of 'fit' between this general periodization and the responses of employing organizations. Thus, the period of the early/mid-80s saw a range of responses by organizations, often negative in their orientation towards people with HIV/AIDS, and aimed at identifying those with, or suspected of, carrying the virus and isolating or excluding them. These attempts were mostly reactive and uncoordinated, responding to notions of threat and panic current in media presentations of the epidemic. Although pressure groups formed by people affected by the disease were making representation to organizations and trying to articulate an appropriate response, these appear to have been relatively limited in their impact at this stage. Thus, the bulk of employers were effectively left to their own devices in responding to the virus. In the ·US there was a particular and widespread concern about the effect that AIDS would have on employee medical insurance policies, but more generally there was, in addition, an outbreak of often indiscriminate sackings and harassment of suspected employees, a response also apparent in Europe where the insurance issue had not assumed the same significance. This discriminatory action was sometimes at the direct instigation of managements, at others it was provoked by the fear and hostility of ordinary employees (with which many managers were prepared to collude). Similarly, there were waves of concern in many public service organizations about the risk of having to deal with patients or clients who might be infected with HIV. Towards the end of this period some major employers began experimenting with the use of HIV testing as a means of screening potential employees for the virus. In most western countries even conservative governments had largely been persuaded by the arguments of the 'liberal' establishment, supported by its medical experts, that universal compulsory HIV testing was both impractical and unethical (Bennett and Ferlie, 1994). As such, employers were not encouraged in this direction (although neither were they explicitly prohibited) and official guidance began to emphasize the introduction of 'AIDS policies' as an alternative means by which employers could combat the fears to which HIV/AIDS might give rise.

Thus, the years of the mid-1980s saw the emergence of moves to spread 'good practice' in relation to employment matters through the use of formal policies — although as we discuss in chapters 2 and 3, the exact meaning of good practice and the detailed content of many policies leaves considerable scope for interpretation. The rationale for this type of project was often to try to alert organizations to the existence of a potentially serious economic problem — in the belief that most employers are motivated to act only by the prospect of losing money — and thereby to stimulate them to develop an AIDS policy and/or provide education and training. If such measures were adopted, it was argued, then costs resulting from legal action taken by employees wrongly dismissed on account of HIV status, or from the adverse reaction of clients or employees leading to lost productivity, could be avoided. Providing a strategic and 'rational' response to the irrational fear of AIDS was presented not just as a humanitarian gesture but also as making 'good business sense' (Arkin, 1994). During this time the 'policy initiative' was also joined by many industry, professional and voluntary bodies which produced codes of practice and model policies for their members, covering both the treatment of employees and/or patients and clients. This period also saw, in the UK, the publication of government guidelines relating to employment practice and the establishment of an 'employers' initiative' within the government supported National AIDS Trust. It should be noted that while these policy *initiatives* attracted considerable attention, the actual adoption of such policy seems to have been restricted in the UK to very large companies and to employers in the public sector (IRS, 1991; IDS, 1987).

Post 1988, as the legitimacy of AIDS as an issue of government concern became consolidated, the propriety of formal responses within the organizational sphere was confirmed by measures which claimed legal or quasi-legal authority. In the US, this period saw the incorporation of people with AIDS into the Americans with Disabilities Act (see, chapter 7 below) and thereby their protection in law within the workplace and labour market. Despite pressure from some quarters for comparable legal protection, no such explicit legislative action was forthcoming from European governments. However, in 1989 the European Council and Ministers for Health of the Member States released a Resolution providing common principles for the 'fight against AIDS'. While this covered a wide range of medical/prevention issues it also included the following statement relating to discrimination:

> Any discrimination against persons with AIDS or HIV-positive persons constitutes a violation of human rights and prejudices an effective prevention policy because of its effects of exclusion and ostracism ... The greatest possible vigilance must therefore be exercised in order to combat all forms of discrimination, particularly in recruitment, at the workplace, at school and as regards accommodation and sickness insurance. With regard, more particularly, to accommodation and private insurance, solutions should be found which *reconcile economic interests with the principle of non-discrimination.* (*Social Europe*, 1, 1990, p. 156; our emphasis)

The significance of the highlighted sentence in the above citation can be noted in passing, for it is within employing organizations that the tension between individual human rights and economic interest is often most clearly focused. Indeed, as will be seen throughout this book, many workplace responses to AIDS are closely connected to this duality and to the interests of power pertaining thereto (see, below). A more specific indication of what this entails is to be found in the United Kingdom Declaration of The Rights of People with HIV and AIDS (p. 2), developed in 1991:

> No person should be barred from employment or dismissed from employment purely on the grounds of their having HIV, or having AIDS or an AIDS-related condition; Employers should ensure that their terms and conditions of employment are such as to enable people with HIV, AIDS, or an AIDS-related condition to continue in their employment, and to do so in a healthy and safe working environment; Employers or their

agents should not perform tests to detect the HIV status of current or prospective employees; in respect of the right to work, the right to privacy, and the right to protection from discrimination, there should be no obligation or requirement upon an individual to disclose to an employer their own HIV status, or the HIV status of another person. (cited in Holmyard, 1993)

In the UK, these ideas have indeed provided the basis for the development of thinking about workplace responses to HIV, but they have done so on what has largely been a piecemeal and voluntary basis and with varying degrees of commitment and significantly different forms of interpretation.

Indeed, although the drive to promote policy and good practice in the workplace has not halted since the mid-1980s, its presentation as a matter of urgency with implications for business efficiency has shifted towards a greater emphasis on sound personnel practice as a means of guarding against contingency rather than necessity. There has also been something of a shift away from the notion that organizations require a separate and distinct policy on AIDS towards the view that AIDS can be incorporated into existing policies such as health and safety, welfare, or equal opportunities. The 'normalization' of the syndrome during this period is reflected in the fact that one of the major initiatives in this area — the National AIDS Trust's *Companies Act* charter which asks signatories to be prepared to declare themselves publicly as models of good employment practice — has succeeded in securing support from major national/international companies. It is unlikely that such open support would have been so easily forthcoming during the periods when AIDS was less well understood, or when the implications looked like being more dramatic and disruptive.

Constraint and Contingency

It does seem, therefore, that the responses to AIDS within the realm of employing organizations does indeed parallel the more general response patterns noted by commentators, and in this respect it is possible to identify in these responses two broad patterns: defensive and constructive. The former defines AIDS as a threat to organizational stability and objectives and calls for more or less sophisticated methods to detect and control those who are perceived to be 'carriers' of the virus. The constructive response rejects the rhetoric of threat and views AIDS as a challenge to an organization's commitment to supporting human rights and equality of opportunity, a challenge to be faced through positive action rather than protectionism (these ideas are developed more fully in chapters 2 and 3 below).

However, although it may be possible to map out a broad sweep of change with apparently chronological qualities (i.e., a move from defensive to constructive responses), it must be remembered that this is, at best, only a trend, and that within the broad sweep there will be considerable variation and, indeed, contradiction. There are within both defensive and constructive responses many different strands, and the boundary between constructive and defensive responses is by no means clear-cut. In particular, detailed responses will vary according to the perceived 'seriousness' of the issues and the formality with which these are addressed in a manner that is likely to be difficult to predict a priori, although factors such as industrial sector, size of organization, workforce composition, organization culture, employment law, and functional responsibility are all likely to act as mediating forces to some extent.

Industrial Sector

In some industrial sectors, for instance, AIDS will be perceived as having greater significance and be more familiar than in others. Thus, in health-care most organizations have policies and procedures for dealing with possible contact with the virus and, especially in hospitals, many staff will have encountered someone with HIV/AIDS. But although organizations in this sector may be familiar with HIV/AIDS as a medical phenomenon, this does not necessarily mean that they will also have addressed it in terms of social or personnel issues. However, the fact that employees of such organizations are charged with providing medical treatment continues to give their possible infection exaggerated importance in the minds of the public and those who claim to speak on its behalf (see, for example, the report in *The People* referred to above).

In manufacturing and non-medical service organizations the significance of HIV/AIDS is less likely to be reckoned in operational terms — as an issue confronting the organization in the course of its normal functioning — but as a personal matter relating to individual employees and deriving from their 'non-work' activities. In this respect its relevance is more likely to be construed in terms of the effect on individual performance, or as an isolated industrial relations problem arising from disruption caused by the actions of employees who, for whatever reason, see themselves to be at risk from the virus.

The distinction between public and private sectors seems also to be of some significance in shaping responses, given the greater prospects for the public sector to have developed policies and provided training for staff. In the public sector, and especially in local authorities, there is a level of exposure and accountability to both central and local political influence that is not experienced by managers in most private sector businesses. Not only may individuals or pressure groups be able to influence policy by enlisting the active support of councillors (Cockburn, 1991, p. 190f), but the ethos of public responsibility and care provision is likely already to have created a space within which the appropriate response to AIDS can be discussed if not resolved:

> Issues such as confidentiality in relation to personal informa-tion, staff training and support, anti-discriminatory function-ing, health and safety, staff and client consultation in decision-making, and policy and guidelines are all matters which are familiar to local authorities. In effect, AIDS has exposed the inadequacies of local authority policy and practice, and has brought about an urgency to examine each of these concerns afresh. (Cotton and Kumari, 1990, p. 213)

Overall, however, the sectoral determination of functional relevance is unlikely to have an exclusively determining effect on response pat-terns. Many organizations in sectors not directly involved in the provision of services concerned with HIV/AIDS have been in the forefront of high profile positive responses to the epidemic. In this respect, other factors may exercise a more powerful influence.

Organization Size

The relevance of organization size can be seen in several ways. For instance, very small organizations are less likely to have 'professional' personnel departments where some knowledge of the virus and its implications may have been gleaned from the professional literature or good practice guidelines. This can compound the tendency for small proprietors to make highly personal and idiosyncratic decisions relating to employees, in the case of HIV/AIDS, perhaps driven by ignorance and/or prejudice, with neither the constraints of policy nor trade union presence that may operate in larger organizations. Similarly, the strongly individualistic and often parochial outlook of many business owners can result in resistance to good practice which is perceived as unwanted outside interference. The financial instability of many small businesses, especially their perceived vulnerability to staff illness, may also lead many to over-react to the threat which they perceive AIDS to represent to their workforces, encouraging dismissal and discrimination at recruitment stages as means of pre-empting this. We have ourselves run awareness courses for small firms where a recurrent concern was to identify and exclude those who might have HIV because they feared incapacity through illness. Ironically, when pressed they expressed no similar concern about any other medical condition, nor did they contemplate the need for medical screening for any illness other than AIDS.

Alternatively, of course, the greater particularism and informality of the small organization can allow greater support for a person affected and for flexibility in deployment, although this is likely to apply more to organizations operating in professional settings than in, say, manufacturing where working practices may have little slack as the result of the need for highly competitive pricing.

Large organizations, of course, are not immune from the exercise of discriminatory behaviour. Bureaucratic procedures may act as a brake upon the exercise of individual prejudice but their very impersonality can lead to the countenance of measures such as HIV testing that appear to have an economic rationality that disguises their human impact. In addition, there is nothing in formal policies or bureaucratic rules *as such* to prevent individuals from behaving repressively. Indeed, in large organizations such behaviour can be both facilitated and concealed by the complex chains of authority and control that distance policy-makers from those supposedly subject to it.

Workforce Composition and Attitudes

The composition of the workforce also seems to play a significant role in shaping responses to the epidemic. The well-publicized stance of Levi Strauss as an organization prepared to make a public commitment to fighting the epidemic and supporting employees affected, originated in its San Francisco headquarters at the instigation of a group of gay employees (Kohl *et al*, 1990). In this respect the existence of a sizeable, articulate and openly gay presence within the local workforce is likely to have had a greater impact in terms of shaping policy than in organizations where homosexuality is neither acknowledged nor accepted as legitimate. Hussey (1995) for instance, recounts the following experience of providing education and training about HIV to a large UK company: 'None of my trainees knew of any openly gay or lesbian employees in the organization (in a workforce of over 4,000); in fact the prospect of anyone coming out at work was so unlikely it was laughable' (Hussey, 1995, p. 345; see, also, Cockburn, 1991, p. 186ff; Green, 1995). Under such circumstances AIDS issues may be kept off the organizational agenda by a combination of homophobic prejudice and fear that to address such matters will raise questions about the 'normality' of 'ordinary' organization members. This may be especially the case in situations where traditional or conservative social attitudes are prevalent (which may result from national, regional, class or ethnic cultures). An example is provided by Gonsiorek (1993):

> Peter had worked for more than 12 years in the technical end of a high tech firm ... His work was respected, and his technical skills were such that the most difficult challenges were often assigned to him. His sexuality was not generally known at work although he had disclosed his sexual orientation to a few close co-workers. His section was reorganized and a new manager was assigned who was a fundamentalist christian. Through the office grapevine this manager discovered Peter's homosexuality, and immediately fired him, stating that it was an infringement of his civil rights and freedom of religion to have to work with a pervert ... Not a single co-worker from the 12 years of employment was willing to assist Peter. (1993, p. 254)

These effects may also be influenced by age and gender profiles, there being at least some evidence to suggest that older people tend to hold less liberal attitudes towards people with AIDS than do younger ones and that women are more tolerant than men (Herek and Glunt, 1991, Green, 1995). Similarly, the occupational structure may have some bearing on responses, particularly the presence of 'professional' grade employees with higher levels of education and awareness (Marquet *et al*, 1995) who might be expected to hold more liberal views towards people with HIV/AIDS.

Organizational Culture

Also bearing upon these types of response is likely to be the organizational culture. Of particular significance are those cultures where a strong emphasis is placed upon issues of employee welfare, employer responsibility and equal opportunities (see chapter 3 below). Belgrave (1995) provides an account of The Body Shop cultural orientation which appears to epitomize this stance:

> The Body Shop is a company committed to the education and empowerment of our employees and to the creation of active citizens in the workplace. As such we are well placed to provide information to our employees on a wide range of issues. We are committed to a high standard of care for our employees ... we try to be like a family in the way we relate to each other, care for each other and celebrate together. The Body Shop is also a company with a young workforce and young customers, many of whom we can assume are sexually active and therefore potentially at risk of HIV infection. Quite simply, we are concerned for the health of our employees. (Belgrave, 1995, p. 357)

Such strong cultures remain relatively unusual among private sector organizations, being most likely to be found in larger companies, and in many other cases cultural dynamics will be driven more by the values of economic and market instrumentality. In the public sector, however, social justice remains (if somewhat less securely now than in the past) a characteristic of many organizations, especially in local authorities where, according to Halford (1992), over half of those in Britain have developed equal opportunities policies. This greater concern is also reflected in the development of specific HIV/AIDS policies where public sector organizations have led the way with 53 per cent claiming to have policies compared to 20 per cent in the private sector (Brodie, 1994. p. 136).

Employment Law

At present in the UK, those areas of employment law which have relevance to AIDS/HIV concern three main issues: discrimination; confidentiality; and dismissal. However, because these areas of law do not deal with HIV/AIDS specifically there is considerable room for contestation and ambiguity. These issues are dealt with fully in chapters 6 and 7 and will not be considered in detail here, except to note that such ambiguity gives considerable room for manoeuvre, especially to employers. In the absence of explicit and clear legal responsibilities, as in the case of, say, sex and race discrimination, many employers are likely to feel that the law places only limited constraints upon their actions in dealing with issues relating to HIV/AIDS. This may be exacerbated by the fact that both parties in a dispute over HIV status can feel they have an interest in, or no alternative to, settling the matter 'informally': the employee to preserve his/her health (and identity) from the stress of litigation, and the employer to be able to 'lose' the employee quickly and quietly with minimum disruption.

Functional Responsibility

In those organizations that develop formal responses to HIV/AIDS the functional specialism of those who take responsibility for framing this response can be of considerable importance. On present evidence it seems that at least three functional areas are closely involved in formulating organizational responses: occupational health; personnel; and trade unions.

Occupational health

In many organizations, especially large ones, responsibility for dealing with matters related to HIV/AIDS is lodged with occupational health practitioners/departments. It is obvious that as HIV-infection will, at some stage, effect a change in an individual's health, it should be a matter for organizational health specialists. Similarly, such specialists can be expected to have expert knowledge of the mechanisms and risks of viral transmission that concern many organization members. The merit of this approach is seen to lie in the assumption that a response grounded in the provision of objective medical 'facts' will allay irrational fears and concerns that people may have about the risk of contracting HIV at work and allow these to be dealt with in an individual, low-key and confidential manner.

This does, however, raise a number of questions. Firstly, it can be suggested that perceptions of risk are not determined solely by possession of objective information (i.e., that those who are well informed will behave rationally, and those who are not, irrationally). Sim (1992), for example, identifies three risk-factors associated with any given hazard — 'magnitude', 'probability', and 'acceptability' — which together contribute to shaping individual responses to that hazard. In relation to HIV/AIDS the factors of magnitude and probability are, in theory, amenable to relatively objective categorization. The *magnitude* of this particular hazard, that is the likelihood of it proving fatal to an individual in contact with it, is known to be high to the extent that the link between contracting HIV, developing related illnesses, and resulting death is strong, albeit of variable duration. However, the *probability* of an individual contracting HIV, especially through occupational activity of any sort, is extremely low as the virus can only be transmitted through exchange of bodily fluids. The third factor — *acceptability* — is of a qualitatively different character in that it relates not to objective or verifiable fact, but to questions of moral choice and subjective judgment. This is especially relevant in the case of HIV/AIDS because it is a disease which is defined not merely through medical and physiological categories, but also through layers of moral meanings, in particular the notions of deviance and homosexuality which have been characterized in much of the media as 'dangerous' and perverse (Lupton, 1994a).

Extending this model to recognize a variable relationship between its components results in at least three possible configurations, each with differing implications for the definition and reaction to perceived risk. A purely *rational response* would assume that individuals are in possession of, and fully accept, accurate information relating to the magnitude and probability of risk and, on this basis, make an informed choice about the level of acceptability they will tolerate. It would thus be expected that the level of acceptability within an occupational context would be high because of the objectively small risk of becoming infected through work related activity. Thus, if properly informed there should be no need for employees either excessively to fear contracting the virus, or to resist working with infected co-workers or clients.

However, as is now well established, individuals do not operate wholly or consistently on the basis of such rational decision-making and, for this reason, it is necessary to consider other possibilities. Thus, the *boundedly rational* response recognizes that individuals often operate with information that is either factually incomplete, incorrect or misunderstood. There is, according to Sim (op cit), a tendency for individuals to assess rare hazards as more common than they actually are, particularly if they have received significant publicity or been presented in a dramatic and vivid manner, and those perceived as 'unnatural' and/or uncontrollable are commonly overestimated. The hazards associated with HIV/AIDS are, therefore, likely to be inflated where attention is focused on the magnitude of the risk without equal attention to the true probability.

Finally, the *Subjective Response* reverses the interpretive connections. Here it is moral or subjective beliefs that determine the level of acceptability which, in turn, serves either to 'reinterpret' magnitude and probability data in line with such preconceptions or to disregard them altogether if they are at variance. For example, the views of a nurse-tutor are quoted by Sim:

> ... frankly, I have no sympathy with homosexuals who contract the disease. This is because it has been contracted through performing an unnatural act — a biological fact. Therefore, while nurses have a duty of care for the sick, we must also recognize that it is 'self-inflicted' in the truest sense of the term, and need not have arisen in the first place. What makes AIDS more horrific is that a stranger's perverse sexual actions can harm totally unknown innocents. (1992, p. 572)

In practice, therefore, individuals are likely to use a complex mix of these decision-making processes in their assessment of risk, the predominance of any one mode depending not only on the accuracy of factual knowledge about the disease, but also attitudes and beliefs about those linked with it, as shaped by personal experience, local cultures and media representation.

A second objection to a narrow occupational health response is that the managerial motivation behind the medicalization of HIV/

AIDS may be less straightforward than is sometimes claimed. It has been suggested (see, IDS, 1993a, p. 2) that such an approach can represent a means by which managements hope to avoid confronting the social and equal opportunities questions that a more wide ranging response might expose. Thus, by defining HIV/AIDS as an issue that is strictly the responsibility of medical experts, the effect and (possibly subconscious) intention may be to 'balkanize' it within a supposedly marginal and politically safe area of organizational activity (see, chapter three below). However, although to define HIV/AIDS as a strictly medical/health issue that can be dealt with purely in terms of rational, scientific information may avoid the need to deal directly with associated equal opportunities issues such as sexual orientation, racism and disability, it does not eliminate their effects and, as such, is likely to be ineffective in dealing with discrimination against people with HIV/AIDS.

Finally, the will to 'contain' HIV/AIDS within a narrow medical/scientific frame may be resisted by occupational health specialists themselves. A recent publication for employers by the Society of Occupational Medicine in the UK, for instance, devotes only one of its four sections to a conventional medical analysis of the condition, the remainder being concerned with matters of employment law and personnel practice (SOM, 1992). In addition, the emergence of the so-called 'new public health' (see, chapter 3 below), which places a greater emphasis on health promotion and the empowerment of individuals to take control of factors affecting their health, is likely to encourage a more explicitly politicized view of illness that challenges the social inequalities associated with medical conditions, thereby further encouraging the breakdown of a narrow medical perspective.

Personnel and human resource management

Where occupational health specialists are not employed, or where a broader framing of HIV/AIDS issues is adopted, crucial aspects of response strategy are likely to be dealt with by personnel specialists. Looked at from this perspective a number of possibilities arise. An emphasis may, for instance, be placed on the establishment of formal procedures designed merely to ensure compliance with employment law and consistency with other personnel practices such as health and safety and sickness policy. This approach is most likely in an environment where the role of personnel has been influenced by a tradition of bureaucratized industrial relations, and where management has accepted a view of employment relations as essentially confrontational and characterized by a need to protect organizational (i.e., management's) interests against the conflicting demands of the workforce. In line with this stance, the approach towards HIV/AIDS will probably be defensive or neutral in the sense that procedural rectitude is designed to protect the organization from problems that might be caused by HIV/AIDS, rather than with providing positive assistance and protections for those affected.

However, where the personnel function has an orientation that is geared more towards the safeguarding of employee interests against the possible excesses of management and promoting equality of opportunity and diversity within the workforce, the approach may come closer to the positive or constructive position. In this respect, more attention will be given to education and attitude-change initiatives in addition to procedural developments designed to prevent discrimination against people with HIV/AIDS and facilitate their continued employment if so desired.

Trade Union Presence

In the UK, many employee concerns related to AIDS have been channelled through trade union representation and reflected on three main dimensions of union policy:

> i) protection from discrimination for those members who may become infected with HIV or develop AIDS;
> ii) measures to limit the possibility of members contracting the virus through their work;
> iii) the provision of information to members concerning the facts about AIDS in order to prevent ignorance damaging employment relationships and to help members contribute effectively to the resolution of any problems that arise in the workplace.

The emphasis given to AIDS has varied between individual trade unions. Perhaps not surprisingly, health service unions were amongst the first to address the implications of AIDS and have continued to give it a high profile as a workplace issue. Taking a wider view, the Trades

Union Congress (TUC) has played a role in the campaign against the spread of HIV since its implications were first recognized in the UK. A 1987 resolution called for, amongst other things, explicit workplace policies on non-discrimination against people with AIDS, the provision of a support and counselling network and a comprehensive education programme on AIDS. The TUC has stated its view of the employment implications of AIDS as follows:

> Many workplace difficulties will be averted by information and a full exchange of views between the parties, backed by agreed, and, where necessary, amended procedures. But such steps must be accompanied by vigilance and the enforcement of health, safety and first aid regimes. The basis of this approach is good practice resting on the moral force of treating people fairly at work. We place heavy emphasis on the fact that in most cases good practice developed for all staff should be applied to people with AIDS in exactly the same way as they apply to people with other potentially life threatening diseases such as heart disease or cancer. This would apply equally in the context of benefit provision if and when employees with AIDS fall sick or become disabled because of the effects of the disease. (Quoted in IDS, 1987, p. 11)

Influences Underlying Contingency

By looking at organizational responses to HIV/AIDS in terms of these contingent factors it is possible to see the potential for detailed variations of reaction and to appreciate that, at any given time, an organization may exhibit elements from different response patterns simultaneously. For example, we may find in the 1990s organizations that are still responding defensively against employees affected by the virus and also companies which have formal policies providing for a constructive response but where, at the level of informal practice, discrimination is still practised.

Thus, despite the diversity that can arise from the interplay of contingent factors, it is also possible to suggest the operation of broad principles that are central to the structuring of employment and organization in contemporary capitalist societies. The most developed of organization structures are rooted in principles of economic rationality emphasizing the need for administrative efficiency and managerial control of both physical and human resources in the pursuit of profit or budgetary targets. Thus, work organization is, to a greater or lesser extent, patterned around principles of hierarchical authority which, *inter alia*, demand the management of labour in the service of objectives determined by the owners/managers of the enterprise. However, this hierarchical structuring is not confined to the purely 'economic' dimensions of organizational life but reflects other 'interests of power', in particular, those constituted around relations of gender, race, sexuality and disability (Cockburn, 1991; Hearn and Parkin, 1994) which create their own gradings of authority, status and opportunity within the organization.

In addition, informal workplace practices cross-cut formal lines of demarcation and differentiation, developing on the basis of associations and commonalities that are facilitated, intentionally or unintentionally, as a result of the divisions of labour that constitute the formal organization. Such practices, however, are not only a response to the conditions of the workplace itself, but rely heavily on the meanings and definitions that members bring with them from outside the organization. So, on the one hand, informal groupings (and associated meaning systems) may develop out of shared situations directly linked to working practices, and often involve the identification and ostracism of outsiders, for example, those who break the informal group's rules, or who are perceived as having conflicting interests to those of the group. However, on the other hand, informal associations often develop around wider societal notions of identity that differentiate some members of a workforce from others, insiders from outsiders: white from black; men from women; straights from gays; disabled from able-bodied. These identities cut across all manner of internal organizational boundaries, as opposed to work role identities that are largely defined by, and exist within, them. Thus, to take but one example, antagonism towards homosexuality may unite straight employees across formal hierarchical divisions to the extent that, despite formal policies outlawing discrimination on the grounds of sexual orientation, the actuality of workplace life is characterized by hate and prejudice towards the outsider group.

In these respects, therefore, it is important to recognize the complex ways in which AIDS is 'organized' within workplace settings, how it is defined and embedded — framed — within formal and informal organizational discourses and how these are constructed, reproduced and challenged through the actions and interactions of organization members. As Collinson (1992) puts it:

> Members of organizations at various hierarchical levels are skilled and knowledgeable actors in both a social and technical sense ... As self-conscious and self-reflexive beings, they constantly try to monitor and make sense of their own behaviour, status and identities, that of 'significant others' and the complex relations between them. Subsequently, they define situations and act in accordance with their definitions in ways that are often self-fulfilling. Human beings in organizations routinely engage in the construction of a meaningful social world through their accounts, relationships, and practices. These constructions of meaning condition, are shaped by and are embedded in the social reproduction of organizational power structures, sub-cultures, personal identities and everyday interactions. (Collinson, 1992, p. 28)

In all these respects, therefore, the nature of workplace organization will play an important role in shaping how the epidemic is experienced, for good or for ill. In the remainder of this book we try to elucidate some aspects of the complex ways in which the meaning of AIDS has been constructed within organizational contexts and has, in turn, (re)constructed the meaning of those contexts.

We begin by developing in chapter 2 an account of the ways in which the definition of AIDS as *general threat* is translated into what we term 'defensive' organizational responses. These can range from crude intimidation and expulsion, initiated not only by employers but also other employees, based on social stereotypes of deviant 'outsiders', to more sophisticated techniques incorporated into policies and personnel practices through which the less favourable treatment of people with HIV or AIDS is legitimated by recourse to the logic of a balance of interests and the greater good.

Chapter 3 moves to an analysis of those responses to HIV/AIDS that define themselves in opposition to the defensive reaction. Constructive responses frame HIV and AIDS as issues that challenge what are assumed to be the underlying humanitarian ethics of organizations in liberal democratic societies — a challenge that can be met with positive policies. There is within these responses a strong dependence on the rhetoric of equal opportunities and, more recently, diversity management and normalization techniques. However, as with other initiatives that have sought to address entrenched inequalities, such strategies are subject to contestation over their objectives — as these invariably involve some level of attack upon embedded interests — and resistance to their implementation in practice. In the case of HIV/ AIDS, it is possible to suggest two areas in which such contradictions and contestations are likely to be articulated and shaped within the context of the workplace.

The first, dealt with in chapter 4, concerns the subjective under-standings which organization members deploy in relation to the epidemic, and how these are framed and reframed within the context of the meanings and motives that guide the conduct of work within employing organizations. It is possible to identify in these subjective understandings a tension between the formal principles of rationality that represent an organization's 'official' or public response to a given situation and the emotionally loaded feelings through which actors experience this and construct an 'appropriate' response. In relation to HIV/AIDS, there emerges a strong sense of uncertainty and apprehen-sion among both those infected with the virus and those who are not, as to the 'right' way to respond within the context of the employment relationship. This seems to reflect the distinction made by Toffler (1986) between moral *issues* ('easy to name', acontextual, widely agreed upon, amenable to simple choice between 'right' and 'wrong') and moral *dilemmas* ('hard to name', context-specific, contentious, complex and conflicting, not amenable to clear judgments). In many respects, the notion of a moral issue fits well the formal organizational response to HIV/AIDS, whereas that of a moral dilemma characterizes how individuals experience the questions and choices which HIV/ AIDS introduces into the conduct of organizational action (Maclagan and Snell, 1992; Goss, 1993). Specific dimensions of these dilemmas are explored in the chapter as are the implications for the relationship between formal policy and workplace practice.

Chapter 5 addresses the second area where the employment implications of HIV/AIDS are crucially shaped, namely, the structuring of sex and gender relations. Most obviously this involves the issue of sexual orientation which has had particular implications within the context of the AIDS epidemic given the tabloid press representation of the disease as 'caused' by homosexual men (Watney, 1987). The result has often been a focusing and accentuating of homophobia within organizations, activated and reproduced through both vertical and horizontal relations. As Gutek (1989, p. 56) has remarked: 'the ... recent spread of AIDS has helped to redefine sexual behaviour at work and elsewhere from being invisible, private and individual to being visible, public and organizational'. In addition, however, the epidemic is also gendered, and it is likely that within the context of employment women will experience its effects differently to men. Finally, it is important to remember that sex work is also a form of employment and one where not only are the risks of HIV transmission real and significant, but also the tensions between the exigencies of earning a living and care of the self, both physically and psychologically, are more acutely experienced.

Chapter 6 moves the debate beyond the bounds of the employing organization and explores the ways in which AIDS has been defined though various dimensions of employment law. Although the interpretation and coverage of legislation is variable it nevertheless provides a formalized rule framework that, to a greater or lesser extent, both limits and facilitates the responses the organizations may develop. In addition, the availability of legal remedy may be one mechanism that offers the possibility of protection to the person with HIV/AIDS within the sphere of employment. The chapter, therefore, outlines the nature of these protections and also their limitations within the UK. One theme which emerges from this analysis is the tendency for the UK legal system to construct the problem of HIV/AIDS in a manner which, in practice, seeks to provide protection for the supposedly uninfected majority from the infected minority.

Finally, chapter 7 extends this analysis into the international sphere by considering comparable issues in European legislative responses to the epidemic and, in particular, The Americans with Disabilities Act.

In these chapters, we are not looking to determine the financial costs of the epidemic to employers or to governments, but rather to explore the relationships, meanings and actions through which responses to HIV/AIDS within the context of employment are constructed, maintained and articulated. Thus, it is not our intention to provide prescriptive models of good practice for employers to adopt. This is not because we feel that 'good practice' is unimportant or undesirable but, rather, because we are acutely conscious that what constitutes good practice is both contentious and contestable, a site for political struggle rather than a standard set of practices that can simply be prescribed. Indeed, one of the key themes of the book will be to demonstrate how numerous attempts to develop forms of good practice in the workplace are underpinned by interests of power and influence that can either compromise or facilitate the employment opportunities and/or life-chances of people with HIV/AIDS and those who have been touched by the epidemic. In our view good practice is not to be taken as given, but rather to be approached critically with a view to exposing the limits of its possibilities within particular settings. It is an understanding of the nature of these limits and the interests which underlie them that should form the basis for strategies of change and development.

Chapter 2

Defensive Responses to HIV/AIDS

Introduction

In broad terms defensive responses, either formal or informal, can be characterized by a distinctive orientation towards HIV/AIDS and to the social repercussions of being infected by HIV. Fundamentally, this involves the assumption that HIV/AIDS poses exceptional human difficulties for the organization, in particular, that employees or clients who carry the virus will, sooner or later, generate problems that will adversely affect organizational performance. These 'problems' can include the fear of cross infection through workplace activity, concern about indirect social disruption caused by the anxiety and prejudice of others, and the consequences of prolonged absence or impaired capacity and associated sickness, insurance or replacement costs.

The hallmark of the defensive response, then, is the perception that HIV/AIDS poses a significant threat to organizational interests and performance which, in turn, supports the need for 'protectionist' measures. The nature and extent of such protectionism, however, is subject to considerable variation, both in terms of driving motives and practical policy measures. Thus, at one extreme, are what may be termed crude or 'direct' defensive responses geared towards the identification and expulsion of the person with, or suspected of having, HIV/AIDS. At the other, are more sophisticated measures where the threat of AIDS is defined as a real but specific rather than universal concern, such that the treatment of the person affected is governed by restrictions on their activities rather than by expulsion. In this instance the logic is of differentiation and regulation rather than automatic removal.

It is arguable that 'sophisticated' defensive approaches represent a reaction to crude practices based on stereotypical prejudice, focusing instead on response patterns that are consistent, standardized and based on the presence of infection rather than the perceived social identity of the carrier. Certainly, most of the approaches falling into this category would claim to be anti-discriminatory in intent, responding benignly to objective scientific information evaluated against the interests of the organization and/or those it represents (clients, patients or employees). Even if this rationalist case is accepted, however, the very definition of HIV/AIDS as a threat about which 'something must be done', establishes a conflict of interests between the organization and the person(s) with HIV/AIDS which it may be difficult for those, charged with safeguarding organization performance, not to resolve in favour of the organization.

In both crude and sophisticated defensive responses, then, the underlying assumption is of the person with HIV/AIDS as an object of threat and suspicion, justifiably subject to control and regulation over and above that applied to 'normal' organization members. There is, in fact, no reason to assume that these responses are necessarily mutually exclusive. For instance, the formal 'safeguards' built into sophisticated responses may easily be over-ridden or ignored by individuals or groups within an organization who, for whatever reason, are determined to avoid any contact with a person with HIV/AIDS, and are prepared to act in an explicitly discriminatory way to achieve this. As will be discussed in the following chapter, this is also a potential problem for constructive responses.

Indeed, to some extent this slippage is probably unavoidable given the complexity of the factors which underlie the fear of AIDS, but the issue is the extent to which defensive responses, even if not necessarily openly encouraging the exercise of prejudice may, nevertheless, implicitly support its practice. A considerable part of this fear is bound up with deep rooted cultural associations with pollution, sexuality and the notion of invasion. As Lupton (1994b, p. 131ff) has pointed out, AIDS has become associated with one of the dominant themes of western public health discourse, namely, the unclean and contaminating nature of sexual fluids, especially when encountered in 'unnatural situations'. This association is both literal — because such fluids can, indeed, carry an infectious and probably deadly virus — and symbolic. In the latter respect the discourse on AIDS, with its frequent use of metaphors of invasion and war reflects deeper cultural understandings through which concern about pollution of the body (Douglas, 1991) mirrors a more general concern about the transgression of social boundaries by 'invaders' (Sontag, 1991, p. 103ff), not least those which regulate sexual mores. In both these respects — that is, literal and symbolic — AIDS stimulates an already developed tendency to regard regulation of the body and its boundaries as a social necessity. Thus:

> The discourse of invasion has wider implications for the ways in which the late capitalist societies view the body. It draws upon discourses which target the body as a site of toxicity, contamination and catastrophe, subject to and needful of a high degree of surveillance and control. According to this discourse, no longer is the body a temple to be worshipped as the house of God: instead it has become a commodified and regulated object which must be strictly monitored by its owner to prevent lapses into health-threatening behaviours. (Lupton, 1994b, p. 134)

In this respect, AIDS has merely accentuated and focused concerns about the regulation of the body that are already apparent in many organizations, especially those where the appearance, functioning, visibility and physicality of employees are perceived to be crucial to the commercial or professional function of the enterprise, for example, medical and social care work, food preparation and serving, etc.

AIDS, Threat and Organization

The threatening discourses of HIV and AIDS mesh easily with the vocabularies of the work organization, especially the private business, where similar metaphors of war, attack, and battle against competitors are commonly evoked and which, in turn, demand the need for defensive strategies and tactics (Shaw, 1990; Knights and Morgan, 1990). In short it is not surprising that in many work organizations, already accustomed to framing new challenges in terms of military metaphors, the encounter with HIV/AIDS should lead to an acceptance of the idea of AIDS as an enemy of the organization — as opposed to a health state of individuals — and lead to the formulation of protectionist responses. In this they have also been able to draw upon traditional ideas of health and illness that continue to inform practices of health and safety at work, where the emphasis is on the managerial duty, in law and good practice, to protect employees and the public from hazard. Thus, when faced by widely circulating discourses of threat, no matter how exaggerated or misinformed, the tendency to over-react by developing defensive measures was and is encouraged on the grounds of 'better safe than sorry'. Parenthetically, it is notable that such measures seem to gain managerial approval with greater ease when their effect is 'merely' to curtail the rights or opportunities of minority social groups, than when they involve financial costs to the organization, such as better plant or more rigorous safety measures.

Thus, traditional infection-management logics, developed in response to easily contagious diseases, have been applied with excessive stringency to a virus that exhibits a very specific and generally low level of infectiousness. These responses can be seen to operate at four levels of intensity that also reflect a move from crude to sophisticated responses:

(i) unilateral expulsion of people with HIV/AIDS based on fear or prejudice;
(ii) pre-emptive attempts to identify and exclude those carrying the virus by the use of HIV testing;
(iii) appeals to self-regulation and voluntary disclosure; and
(iv) frameworks of rules established through formal policy.

Unilateral Expulsion

This response operates on the basis of a perceived imminent threat such that the identification of those considered to be 'viral vectors' becomes a key concern (Wilson, 1994). Thus, attention tends to focus on either the social stereotypes held to be responsible for the spread of infection and/or on an exaggerated conception of the virus as highly infectious, even contagious. For example, attempts to exclude from organization membership those perceived to belong to so-called high risk groups may be motivated by deep-rooted personal prejudice against group members' presumed lifestyle such that contracting HIV/AIDS is seen as further compounding an already deviant status; certainly, surveys of the difficulties faced by homosexual employees support the view of significant levels of discrimination based on sexual identity (Jury, 1993; Diamant, 1993). Alternatively, exclusion can result from an apparently amoral strategic calculation that organizational interests are best served by adopting a discriminatory approach. This latter position is at least partially illustrated by an Equal Opportunities Commission (EOC) investigation into the practices of Dan Air in 1987 (see, also, chapter 6 below) where a policy of not recruiting male stewards appears to have been adopted with the sole purpose of avoiding the employment of gay men:

> At the time of the [EOC] investigation, Dan Air admitted a policy of recruiting only women for cabin-crew posts. This was direct discrimination against men and therefore contrary to the [Sex Discrimination] Act. The airline said that it had a defence under the Health and safety Act, 1974, which permitted it to select women rather than men. It said that over 30 per cent of the men applying for jobs were gay. As AIDS mainly affects homosexuals there was a risk of infection if male staff had an accident aboard the plane . . . The EOC obtained evidence from two senior doctors which suggested that there was no health risk to passengers. (Harris, 1990, p. 94)

Nonetheless, documented instances of this crude defensive response in the UK are not legion, although it seems likely that official reporting significantly understates the actual cases. Thus, despite the existence of certain legal safeguards, discrimination against those affected by HIV/ AIDS is not difficult for many employers. On the one hand, UK employment law effectively removes protection from those who have not been employed with the same employer for two or more years or are engaged in part-time work and, as such, is likely to place greater limitations on younger employees — that is, those most likely to have contracted HIV — who may be changing jobs frequently or just entering the labour market. On the other hand, there is the distinct possibility that someone with HIV and especially AIDS-related illness, will be unwilling to take their case to a public and uncertain tribunal hearing either for fear of disclosure of their health status, or because they are too ill. These issues have been most fully investigated by Wilson (1992) who draws attention to the clear contradiction between the small number of people who invoke formal legal action — in the UK up until 1991 only six employment law cases mentioned HIV, while the number of enquiries regarding employment rights made to THT and Immunity Law Centre totalled over 2,000 in 1991 alone. She concludes:

> ... every single factor for the generally low use of the law ... will apply doubly to people affected by HIV. If the law is stressful for a healthy person, the stress for someone affected by HIV is likely to be even higher. If the law is too costly for people with a normal life expectancy, one might expect people living with HIV or having progressed already to AIDS will often feel their time is too precious to spend on lengthy and stressful legal action. If the law is generally too public, the burden of that publicity for someone socially stigmatized because of HIV infection will be even greater. (Wilson, 1992, p. 19)

Cases discovered by Wilson include those of a building worker, found to be a previous drug user, whose colleagues refused to work with him unless he had an HIV test. He refused to take a test because he feared he would be dismissed if found to be positive, but was sacked the following week. There was no legal redress as he had not worked for the firm for the minimum two year period. Similarly, a wages clerk with haemophilia who, because bleeding tended to occur in his knees and ankles, had always been allowed to deliver wages to company outlets by car, had this 'privilege' withdrawn when his diagnosis of HIV sero-positivity became known to his employer. Having to deliver the wages on foot, he experienced severe bleeds which resulted in absence from work and eventual dismissal from his job on grounds of ill-health.

In addition to expulsion and exclusion from the workplace, crude defensive responses may also involve the segregation, both physical and symbolic, of those thought to be infected with HIV. In some cases this may result from a genuinely held belief that physical contact with the person or with objects touched by them poses a real threat of infection. But in others this rationale is doubtless invoked to conceal or rationalize a psychological repugnance induced by the presumed identity of the person with HIV/AIDS, or to legitimate forms of social closure directed against those identified as outsiders. Barbour (1994, p. 149), for instance, recounts being told stories of hospital staff 'over-reacting by dressing up in "spacesuits", leaving yellow polythene bags outside rooms, hanging up notices on doors saying "Isolated", supplying separate crockery or cutlery and making provision for separate toilet arrangements' for patients with AIDS.

Indeed, the issue of physical contact has figured in several cases of discrimination against people with, or suspected of carrying HIV, the perceived risk from sharing objects that have been handled and presumably contaminated by an infected person having frequently been cited as cause for expulsion (see, chapter 6 for examples). Claims from other groups of workers for separation from people with HIV can also be found in the police and prison services. A senior UK police officer, for example, has claimed that 'officers and civilian staff run a daily risk of being exposed to deadly viruses from infected prisoners who turn violent', citing the case of a cell matron bitten by a prisoner who said she was HIV positive and reporting that some officers wanted a change in the law to bring in a register of HIV carriers (*Southern Evening Echo*, 28 January, 1993 p. 3). Similarly, until 1992 Wandsworth prison (London) had a policy of segregating prisoners known to carry HIV, isolating them in a special unit, leading to claims that these prisoners were being stigmatized and denied rights and facilities available to other prisoners. Attempts to move some of these prisoners to normal conditions in other jails were initially resisted by prison officers, although by late 1992 the unit had been closed, its inmates dispersed and claims made that all new arrivals with HIV would be treated as 'ordinary prisoners' (Carvel, 1992).

This type of response is not aimed only at people who are known to be infected with HIV or who are assumed to fit the stereotype of a so-called risk-group member. They can also be seen in relation to the reactions encountered by people involved in AIDS-related work, as Barbour (1993) recounts:

> ... folk — even people we've worked with before — just cutting you dead now because you work in the AIDS [unit] ... because they disapprove of us working with drug users, I suppose ... 'Once we'd been visiting a friend. And when I went to leave this bloke said to me (he'd asked me what I'd worked at), he said, "Now you just smash that glass you've drunk out of before you leave, because I'm certainly not going to use it again".'
> (Barbour, 1993, pp. 163–62)

Cockcroft, however, provides a clear example from medical practice where perceived social identity did serve as a basis for differentiation:

> ... the approach of identifying HIV-infected patients is in fact neither logical nor effective. It can lead to bizarre anomalies as staff make decisions based on what they know or suspect about a patient's HIV status, rather than on blood contamination

potential of the procedure they are undertaking. For example, I have seen staff washing down the walls of operating theatres after non-bloody procedures on HIV positive patients, while other staff repeatedly changed a patient's tracheotomy tube without wearing gloves because they knew he had a girlfriend and so thought him unlikely to be HIV positive (in fact, he was HIV antibody positive). (Cockcroft, 1991, p. 7)

Ironically, the use of HIV testing within the context of employment has been justified by many of its proponents as much on the grounds that it prevents this type of social prejudice and misjudgment as on its crude exclusionary function.

Workplace Testing for HIV

The use that is made of HIV testing by work organizations, while by no means common, represents a more sophisticated and, apparently, objective method of responding to HIV/AIDS. In general, it has been presented by its proponents as a strategy designed to protect an organization against significant and unreasonable costs or disruption that would be posed by a person with HIV. Alternatively, in the context of medical and social care organizations testing has been argued to offer a means of protecting staff and patients from the risk of accidental infection. In some cases, testing is also justified on the grounds that a positive result enables a person to be given better protection or care, in the case of hospital staff, for example, by not exposing them to stressful jobs or work with contagious diseases. Despite these apparently benign intentions and the growing recognition of the value of voluntary testing for those who suspect they may have been exposed to the virus (see, for example, Patton 1990), testing within the context of the employment relationship and/or under conditions of heavily constrained or limited choice, remains highly contentious (Pierret, 1992). Thus, although the number of organizations adopting HIV testing appears to remain small, the issues raised are of considerable importance and need to be thoroughly aired if 'knee-jerk' calls for the introduction of workplace testing in the wake of periodic 'panics' are to be resisted, or if this form of testing is not to be introduced into workplace health checks 'by the back door' (see, below).

In terms of the interests of those who control employing organizations testing offers certain apparent benefits as a regulatory technology. In many cases its use has been justified on the grounds of direct cost: employees who fall ill as a result of AIDS will be unproductive or will present a disproportionate drain on resources such as insurance premiums or sick pay; it is thus in the interests of the organization, and its 'healthy' employees for such people to be excluded if possible. For instance, the following examples are cited in a Panos report:

> The [London UK] Metropolitan police in common with other large organizations on a tight budget are looking for people who are likely to give long, effective and regular service. As an employer, we have the right and the duty to ensure this. Since a substantial proportion of people who are HIV positive may go on to develop AIDS, we cannot take the economic risk of employing anyone who is known to have tested positively.

> The Swiss insurance company, La Neuchateloise, requires future employees to be tested, on the grounds that employees are insured by the company itself and the costs incurred by people with AIDS are very high. A similar policy on the grounds of high insurance costs is in force in a British subsidiary of Texaco. (Panos, 1990, p. 66)

In other cases, the concern may be to limit indirect costs such as those that could result from the disruption caused by other employees refusing to work with someone with AIDS, or from lost custom through fear of infection.

In some airlines companies, for instance, the use of HIV testing is part of extensive pre-employment medical checks and is justified, firstly, on the grounds that a person infected with HIV would be putting themselves at risk because of the unpredictable and arduous nature of the work and, secondly, that the chance of AIDS-related dementia would put safety of aircraft at risk (SOM, 1992, p. 24). It should be noted, however, that instances of dementia associated with HIV infection are extremely rare, less than five per cent in people with HIV and less than 20 per cent in people with AIDS, and then only when extremely ill (Harris, 1990, p. 103).

There is also an issue over the practical validity of testing for HIV in relation to employment, over and above the accuracy of the test itself, resulting from the fact that the presently available test identifies antibodies to the HIV virus that are undetectable for up to three months after contracting the virus. Thus, it is quite possible for an individual to contract the virus, to be tested shortly after this and to get a negative result. Alternatively, of course, someone could be correctly tested as being free of the virus, but contract the virus by engaging in, say, unsafe sex immediately after the test. In these regards, therefore, if the purpose of testing is to identify the presence of the virus in employees, then it can only be effective if it is repeated on a regular basis, say at least every year, and not merely on a pre-recruitment basis.

This, of course, raises the possibility that for many of the organizations that engage in testing the intention may be to encourage a form of 'self-selection' whereby those who may feel themselves to have been exposed to the virus, decide not to apply for jobs that involve having to take a test.

The issue of choice is clearly crucial. There are regimes where being tested is a mandatory requirement of employment. Under these conditions the individual clearly does not arrive at the decision to be tested of their own volition and, while they can refuse to submit to the test, this will, almost inevitably, deny them the opportunity of employment. Indeed, in some cases it appears that testing may be conducted covertly or under coercion. A case which came to light in 1994 suggests that employers may decide to undertake testing for HIV without fully informing staff, incorporating it into other medical screening. According to a newspaper report by Dodd and Nelson (1994), over 100 of Harrods' food hall staff were told that they would be required to undergo medical tests, including screening for HIV, following an outbreak of food poisoning. It is claimed that many workers were angry about this but did not complain because they were afraid that they would be sacked, although one chef is launching a test case against the store and another employee has resigned (see, chapter 6 below):

> A kitchen worker, who said her concerns about having the tests were brushed aside by [the company doctor] ... said her blood was taken while she was asking for counselling. 'He put the needle in while we were talking. He said it was not necessary to sign a consent form to have an HIV test.' (Dodd and Nelson 1994)

In organizations where the minimal requirements of a code of practice are not adhered to, there is certainly scope to cause psychological damage as cases reported to Terrence Higgins Trust (THT) and National AIDS Trust illustrate. For example:

> [THT] were contacted by Bill who had been refused a job with a British airline. He was very distressed when he arrived at our offices, because he had been told that he was antibody positive. A few weeks earlier Bill had applied for a job to be an air steward. He was offered the job subject to a medical. He attended the medical at the employer's medical centre where they took some blood. Some weeks later Bill received a letter. It said that he had not passed the medical as the tests carried out revealed an abnormality in his blood. Distressed by this news he telephoned the centre asking them to explain what they meant by 'abnormality' ... [He was eventually] told he was antibody-positive. Bill was devastated. (Harris, 1990, p. 97)

Equally important is the symbolism and meanings which the imposed HIV test can solidify. As Sontag (1991) has pointed out, the widely held belief that HIV infection is an inevitable death sentence means that a test result can define a person, even if asymptomatic, as already moribund in the eyes of managers or colleagues:

> The obvious consequence of believing that all those who 'harbour' the virus will eventually come down with the illness is that those who test positive for it are regarded as people-with-AIDS, who just don't have it ... yet. It is only a matter of time, like any death sentence. Less obviously, such people are often regarded as if they *do* have it. Testing positive for HIV ... is increasingly equated with being ill. Infected *means* ill, from that point forward ... Being ill in this new sense can have many practical consequences. People are losing their jobs when it is learned they are HIV-positive ... and the temptation to conceal a positive finding must be immense. (Sontag, 1991, p. 118)

Such a belief is made almost inescapable by the use of testing as a differentiating and exclusionary device, as opposed to a means of facilitating individual control over a potential illness. And as such it has the power to legitimize any reluctance to hiring people with HIV/AIDS, even if it is accepted they pose no threat to others, on the grounds that their imminent incapacity will result in financial cost, either in terms of replacement, or lost training investment. It also supports a disempowering conception of the person with HIV/AIDS, defined as someone with no viable future career and little contribution to make towards organization performance. In short, to sustain the viability of testing at the point of entry it is necessary to construct an image of the person with HIV/AIDS as a potential threat; and although this may not be articulated explicitly through the crude language of social deviancy, the rationalistic balance of imminent incapacity and death against organizational costs is no less destructive and dehumanizing in its effects.

Indeed, testing also symbolises the stance of the organization regarding the bodily attributes and behaviours of its desired workers. In this respect it not only affects potential employees who may be subjected to it, but also acts as a discipline for those already in employment, even if they themselves do not have to undergo the test. This is not so much a discipline that explicitly stops employees engaging in behaviours that may put them at risk of infection, but rather one which regulates identities. By explicitly prohibiting people with HIV/AIDS as organization members it implicitly outlaws those identities that have become associated with it such that individuals are likely to suppress these for fear that they will be subject to sanction through 'AIDS-association'. As Sontag (op cit, p. 110) puts it:

> to get AIDS is precisely to be revealed, in the majority of cases so far [in the western industrial nations] as a member of a certain 'risk group', a community of pariahs. The illness flushes out an identity that might have remained hidden from neighbours, jobmates, family, friends.

Disclosure and the Need to Know

As already stated, the use of testing as a routine screening mechanism has not been widely used by UK organizations. More common has been the practice of requiring, or encouraging, employees to self-disclose their actual or suspected antibody status to the organization, either at the point of recruitment or at any time subsequently. IDS (1993a) report the following procedure adopted by a major UK-based multinational company:

As part of these [medical] examinations, it is normal company practice to request applicants and employees to inform the examining medical officer of various illnesses they may have had. Applicants and employees will be expected to make known if they have good reason to believe that they have been infected with HIV. Information disclosed to company medical officers is always treated by them in strictest confidence and disclosure of infection with HIV will be no exception ... An employee's service with the company will not normally be terminated solely on the basis of having become infected with HIV. If ill health does result, a decision regarding continued employment will be made as in any other case of illness. (IDS, 1993a, p. 15)

Two general issues are raised by this type of approach. The first concerns the apparent equation of HIV infection with having had an illness. The implied message here is the organization's concern with impending and inevitable incapacity, rather than with the actual capability of the infected-but-well employee. The use of a term like 'good reason to believe' also raises questions about its purpose, seeming to cover not only the actuality of infection, if known, but also whether the person has engaged in presumed high-risk behaviour — a concern that goes beyond the medical and towards a normative judgment of lifestyle. These implications problematize the accepted notion of 'fitness for employment' at the time of the medical examination as the normal criteria for appointment (SOM, 1992, p. 27). Indeed, given that people may live with HIV for more than twenty years without debilitating illness, the very utility of *needing* to know HIV status at the asymptomatic stage must be called into question, certainly for employment where there is no risk of infection to others — virtually all jobs outside of medical practice — and where wholly extraordinary demands are not made on the body.

Secondly, there are issues concerning the form that disclosure takes. In particular, the common usage of self-administered questionnaires can raise questions of confidentiality if administered by a personnel department rather than a company doctor. In our experience, personnel departments often have significantly different understandings of confidentiality from medical professionals. In the former case it usually means that the information does not go formally beyond the department, but there may be little notion of confidentiality within the department itself. Here such questionnaires may form part of an employee's general personnel record and be made available to any manager requiring them for purposes such as appraisal or grievance (for a related incident see, Lesslie, 1994). The most formalized mode of disclosure and probably the strongest case for an employer's need to know is associated with employment in the health sector. As an alternative to pre-entry testing, the guidance for UK health care workers provides an ostensibly voluntary code of practice which emphasizes the benefits for the individual. This voluntarism has so far been maintained, despite substantial media coverage of a number of 'infected health worker' incidents, on the grounds that more effective regulation can be achieved by encouraging employees to be tested under conditions of support than by risking 'driving those with the disease underground' because of their fear of the consequences of a positive test result.

Here the discourse of professional responsibility as a form of self-regulation is brought strongly into play. These guidelines are summarised by Mulholland thus:

> ... the General Medical Council states that: 'It is imperative ... that any doctors who think that there is a possibility that they may have been infected with HIV should seek appropriate diagnostic testing and counselling and, if found to be infected, should have regular medical supervision. They should also seek specialist advice on the extent to which they should limit their professional practice in order to protect their patients.' HIV positive doctors are also to act on that advice and this may involve not practising or limiting their practice in certain ways; they are not to rely solely on their own assessment of the risk to patients. Further, where a doctor has counselled a professional colleague infected with HIV to modify his or her professional practice so as to safeguard patients, and is aware that this advice is not being followed, that doctor has a *duty* to inform *an appropriate body* that the colleague's fitness to practice is impaired. (Mulholland, 1993, p. 81)

In 1992/3, following a series of 'scares' involving doctors and surgeons with HIV, Department of Health guidelines confirmed the duty of professional responsibility regarding testing to the extent that, if they think they are infected, health care workers 'must seek advice *and* HIV test where appropriate. Health care workers should be in no doubt about their ethical and professional responsibility' (Virginia Bottomley, cited in DORA, 1993, p. 12). In addition, health authorities have a duty to notify patients and offer them HIV tests if they have received invasive treatment from an infected health worker, although the identity of that worker must be kept confidential from the public and the media. However, this confidentiality can be breached where a GP or occupational physician (OP) is treating a health worker known to be HIV positive and still performing invasive techniques. Under such conditions the GP/OP must report that person to his/her employer and their professional regulatory body (Mulholland, op cit, p. 83).

There remains, however, something of a contradiction between the official position of 'no danger of infection' on the one hand, and the need to establish and widely publicize 'hotlines', letters and counselling on the other. This has been highlighted by DORA (1993):

> If there is so little risk, then it should not be necessary for health authorities and hospital trusts in the United Kingdom to write to patients in such circumstances or to set up special helplines. A senior manager, preferably at the Department of Health must ensure that the actions reflect the words they currently undermine. No letters should be written or helplines established if the risk is so low. (ibid)

This contradiction may be reflected in the distrust which some health workers seem to show towards their management's ability to manage cases of HIV/AIDS. It seems that despite the logic of benign and tolerant understanding embodied in official guidelines, many workers in the health sector are frequently far from certain that their employers, perhaps under pressure from the media, will fulfil the commitment to redeployment and employment protection in practice. Consider, for example, the following anonymous letter to a newspaper from a doctor which illustrates the operation of such 'low trust dynamics' (Fox, 1974):

> If I became HIV positive as a result of what would be an industrial accident, I could predict the outcome. I would be told that the health authority bore no responsibility, as I must have failed to follow 'guidelines' ... I would have to cease practising in my chosen specialty. I have trained for 12 years, working ridiculous hours, passed post-graduate specialist

exams, and written an academic thesis. If lucky I might get moved to a 'low risk' specialty as a junior again. At best I would face a significant cut in income and have to retrain. I suspect the chances of receiving compensation for the loss of my livelihood would be negligible. No doubt it would be implied that the infection occurred outside work. (anon, 1993)

Regardless of the accuracy, or efficacy, of these views they give a clear insight into the perceived consequences of HIV infection for health workers, and allow some understanding of why an infected employee may be reluctant to disclose their antibody status.

Indeed, despite the media attention that has focused on the possible risk caused by infected health workers, there have also been calls, less well publicized, from health workers themselves for the adoption of defensive procedures to protect them from patients infected with HIV. A study of consultants and medical students at a London hospital (Elford and Cockcroft, 1991, p. 154), for instance, found that 'contrary to official medical advice, a substantial proportion of consultant staff and students ... supported compulsory HIV antibody testing of patients.' A survey of US nurses (N=1140) by Lippman (1992, p. 29) revealed that 51 per cent supported the idea of mandatory testing of patients on admission to hospital, and that 82 per cent felt that health care workers had a right to know the HIV status of a patient. This feeling is reflected more forcefully in another section of the anonymous letter quoted above: 'At our hospital the HIV status of patients who receive tests is known by management but not by those of us responsible for treatment, the insulting assumption being that, other than being able to take greater care to protect ourselves, we will treat them differently' (Anon, 1993). The certainty that different treatment will not result, however, cannot be taken for granted. At least one nurse has been struck off the professional register for refusing to treat an AIDS patient, 37 per cent of a survey of UK nurses (cited in Walsh, 1992) believed that they should be allowed to refuse to care for a patient with AIDS, and 27 per cent supported the view that a patient with AIDS should be nursed in isolation from other patients (see, also, Sim, 1992 and chapter 4 below).

This tension between threat and concern, however, is not only found within the context of interpersonal caring relationships, but is also apparent in the constitution of many of the written HIV/AIDS policies adopted by a range of organizations.

From our own analysis of policy documents, all obtained between 1992–94, although many date back to the late 1980s, it is possible to distinguish those which appear to be informed by defensive principles. Twenty-two policies were examined in the original, and a further 30 from secondary sources. Of these, the ratio of Defensive to Constructive (see, chapter 3) is in the order of 1:5. This may be a reflection of a greater preparedness of organizations with Constructive policies, knowing these to be 'good practice', to allow outside disclosure. The basis for our analysis of policy documents is the distinction between two dimensions of content: *conditionality*, the extent to which the treatment of those with AIDS/HIV is conditional upon and subordinate to explicit concerns for organizational interests, either reputation or commercial; and *exclusion*, the extent to which it is regarded as possible or desirable to identify and separate those with HIV/AIDS either by severance/non-employment or by less favourable treatment. Thus, defensive policies have a high degree of both conditionality and exclusion, their objective seeming to be to retain the maximum room for legal manoeuvre for the organization and the protection of its interests, often at the expense, ultimately, of those with HIV/AIDS. These policies, implicitly or explicitly, emphasize the potential risk to the organization of employing or continuing to employ someone with AIDS/HIV, and prioritize this as the key managerial concern. The following analysis is based on extracts from the group of defensive policies, all from the private sector and all from different policies.

Although these policies have a stated concern to deal fairly with employees who are 'AIDS sufferers' (*sic*) they also contain the defensive assumption that HIV/AIDS poses a threat to workplace operations. This is often evidenced in references to the damage which could befall the organization should its managers inadvertently contravene employment laws or generate 'bad publicity', although the emphasis is, tellingly, on the consequences of being 'caught out' rather than the ethical nature of the action itself.

Typically the section which forms the opening text of the policy document and ostensibly sets the tone for that which is to follow, outlines the organization's stance in relation to cases of HIV/AIDS. This statement normally claims its authority from 'senior medical advisors' or from government, and affirms the view that as HIV/AIDS does not pose any appreciable risk within a workplace context, discrimination against people affected will be not tolerated. For example:

> AIDS is a medical condition which has attracted widespread publicity and ill-informed alarm. The government is conducting a major campaign in how the disease is transmitted ... As a result the [organization] has prepared a policy on AIDS which insists on non-discrimination and confidentiality for carriers and sufferers.

As the text of the policy develops, however, a shift of emphasis is often apparent whereby a series of conditions and uncertainties are introduced which, in effect, subtly modify the apparently unconditional meaning of the opening sections. Consider the following illustrations (emphasis added in all cases below):

> Suspension or dismissal solely on the grounds that an employee has become infected is not considered a *practicable* course of action.

> [Managers] are advised to contact their Personnel department for advice *before contemplating* making a job offer to an AIDS carrier.

> Should an applicant be identified at recruitment as being an AIDS victim or virus carrier, discretion will need to be used as to whether the person should be engaged — depending upon the position being sought, general site circumstances or *other sensitivities believed to be likely to have a bearing on the decision.*

Once established this sense of uncertainty and implicit threat serves as the basis for another shift into a mode which establishes the potential for differential treatment of people with AIDS. For example:

> An employee carrying the HIV virus will be considered for any appointment.... subject to the same conditions as would apply to any other applicant. The employment prospects of an *employee suffering from AIDS are so limited that such a person would not be considered a suitable candidate for promotion* ... applications from people suffering from AIDS will not be considered since

their work performance and attendance would be *adversely affected by their condition as to make them unsuitable for employment.*

This, in turn, provides for a further 'shunt' supporting the propriety of surveillance and vigilance:

> In circumstances where it comes to the attention of the unit manager that it is *suspected/*confirmed that we are employing a *potential AIDS suspect,* he/she should immediately notify the Operations Manager. The OM should notify his General Manager Operations, who in turn should notify Personnel and the Regional Director. The RD is responsible for notifying the Divisional Operations Director.

> Should you have any *fears arising from the behaviour or state of health of any of your fellow employees,* you must immediately discuss the matter with your immediate superior.

These reframings 'hang together' because they are written using a vocabulary which establishes and reinforces the 'abnormal' nature of AIDS, reflected in the repeated use of words such as 'victim', 'sufferer', 'carrier' and 'suspect'. In one case this extended to attributing 'responsibility' for the spread of the disease to certain groups and placing these in opposition to their luckless 'victims', but even here the use of words such as 'consort' and 'indulge' suggest that such 'victims' have at least contributed to their own downfall:

> It can be seen that 90 per cent [of AIDS cases] occurred in male homosexuals, the remainder in those injected with infected blood or the unlucky females who consorted with infected bisexuals ... There is no risk of our employees contracting AIDS unless they indulge in sexual intercourse with a male homosexual.

There is, however, an additional strand which can be seen as providing the basis for the various meanings described above. It is this that, ultimately, acts as the 'master frame', the arbiter of the conditions upon which such distinctions are made: namely, the commercial interests of the organization. Thus:

... in general the company will not dismiss an employee purely on the basis he/she has become infected ...

At this stage medical tests for AIDS are not considered appropriate, unless required by legislation or exceptional *commercial contract arrangements...*

To dismiss an individual who is infected or thought to be infected, because of pressure from work colleagues or the client, may expose us to an *unfair dismissal claim, and furthermore to potentially adverse publicity.*

In order *to protect our trading position* against the risks which can stem from public ignorance and alarm, the PR aspects of individual cases will require careful handling. The prime aim will be to eliminate or at worst minimize publicity in each case. If publicity is unavoidable, the PR department should be asked to advise.

Should it become known to management that an employee is carrying the HIV virus or suffering from AIDS this information will be held in the strictest confidence and will be made known only to such others as need to know ... and only with the employee's permission, *except where, permission being withheld, Management concludes, after proper consideration of all the circumstances ... that disclosure is necessary in the best interests of the employee, other employees, or the Company.*

This, then, can be treated as the underlying rationale for this type of policy. Although not spelled out directly, the commercial interests of the organization, as defined by management, provide the basis upon which successive meanings are built. Thus, although the opening statements construe the primary purpose of policy as the protection *of* employees affected by AIDS, most of the substantive content is constructed to suggest the need to protect the organization *from* such persons. In this respect the policies are capable of carrying a dual meaning, either one of which may be 'picked up' by different readers, depending on their interests. When read by an audience not responsible for actually implementing the policy, for example, external observers, junior employees, it may convey the impression that the principal concern is the protection of people with HIV/AIDS. However, for those who are charged with implementing this policy, that is, managers, it is more likely to be interpreted as suggesting a position that is highly conditional and open to transformation.

Thus, although the policy does not prescribe a top-down sovereign power it does operate through the construction of individual choices and tensions which implicitly suggest the 'responsible' solution to the 'problem' that HIV/AIDS is perceived to create. To do other than accept this 'responsible solution' would be to contravene the established normative code of the business organization, that is, the primacy of commercial interest.

Conclusions

This chapter has brought together a number of documented responses that appear to illustrate the definition of the person with AIDS as a more or less serious threat to organizational performance and from which it must be protected. The concern has been the tendency for many forms of organization to seek means of regulating, either by exclusion or seclusion, people with HIV or AIDS who fall within its sphere of control. The motivating force for these regulatory strategies is not necessarily a self-conscious desire to oppress those affected by HIV — although this may be an effect — but more likely to be a protectionist response to what is perceived to be a threat to the objectives and success of the organization or to the safety of certain organization members.

What we have termed the defensive response to HIV/AIDS can be viewed at one level as a form of crisis management strategy through which organization decision makers strive to address what is perceived to be a threat (Pettigrew, Ferlie and McKee, 1992). The characteristics of this form of crisis-as-threat management are outlined by Pettigrew *et al* (op cit) as including: 'increased centralization and formalization, with a breakdown of integrating structures; the erosion of information channels; the exiting of key human resources [e.g., senior managers]; a loss of trust and loyalty as a low commitment organization emerges; groupthink and scapegoating' (1992, p. 109). It should be remembered, however, that for most organizations, that is, excluding those directly involved in the management of AIDS treatment, this crisis has been more anticipated than actual. Thus, although many organizations have had to deal with clients or employees affected by HIV, this has not affected human resource strategies on anything like the epidemic and catastrophic scale anticipated by many commentators in the early 1980s. To this extent it would be surprising to find evidence of all aspects of the crisis management symptoms outlined above and, indeed, the dominant strand of the defensive response seems to have concentrated on the processes of centralization and formalization and/or of groupthink and scapegoating. This appears to have been shaped by, on the one hand, the current media and medical prognosis of the likely spread of the virus and its effects, including dominant stereotypes and prejudices and, on the other, traditional human resource management techniques of tighter regulation, control and policy development. To this extent the response is largely reactive and conservative in form.

Indeed, as the perceived crisis has essentially evaporated for most organizations (as opposed, of course, to individuals), active defensive responses have also apparently been suspended. This does not mean, however, that defensive responses have necessarily been replaced by a more constructive and compassionate approach resulting from greater knowledge and understanding of the disease. It may be more appropriate to think of them as having become latent and, as such, a resurgence of panic about HIV/AIDS — which is quite possible if heterosexual infection rates rise sharply or if homophobic and racist prejudice escalates — may well see many organizations re-engaging with the types of regulatory and defensive responses discussed.

Chapter 3

Constructive Responses to HIV/AIDS

Introduction

Although emerging simultaneously with defensive responses, what we term the constructive response presents a very different orientation towards HIV/AIDS and its organizational consequences. The approach starts from the assumption that either because of its association with stigmatized groups, or simply as a result of its new and apparently implacable potency, HIV/AIDS serves as a basis for, or a justification of, discriminatory behaviour. In particular, constructive responses have been born out of a concern on the part of organization policy-makers to remedy or avoid any form of discrimination in employment, a response usually initiated through an existing commitment to equal opportunities. Alternatively, this response has also been introduced by the efforts of groups organized by, or in support of, people with HIV/AIDS — in particular, but not exclusively, the homosexual community. In this respect the formulation and adoption of constructive responses has been shaped to a considerable extent by the interplay of a number of ideological positions that have emerged in the wake of the epidemic. This has been discussed by Bennett and Ferlie (1994) within the context of the health service, although the ideological forms they identify can, we suggest, be seen as influential in shaping a wider range of organizational responses to HIV/AIDS.

Bennett and Ferlie (op cit) posit the operation of four ideological perspectives on HIV/AIDS: conservative, liberal, professional and radical. It is the last three, however, that have a direct bearing on the constructive response which, in general, can be regarded as a reaction to the conservative ideology which emphasizes moral disapproval towards those with HIV/AIDS and calls for their control and repression (Bennett and Ferlie, 1994, p. 65f; Herek and Glunt 1991).

The *liberal ideology*, according to Bennett and Ferlie, reflects what may best be described as the outlook of the 'Establishment' elite — such as top civil servants, senior managers of public institutions and the old universities — who, they argue, 'wanted to make the country a freer and happier place, and greater personal and sexual freedom was an important part of their agenda' (1994, p. 61). In consequence they contributed to constructing an official definition of AIDS as 'just another disease'. This stance reflected the desire, firstly, to present the state as both compassionate and liberal; secondly, to bring the issue of AIDS under the policy control of its own trusted managers, such as senior civil servants and managers in the Department of Health; and thirdly, to 'head off attempts to introduce massive control measures' that would not only undermine the liberal cause in general but also the 'private' sexual and lifestyle freedoms enjoyed by its own members and supporters (ibid).

Certainly official guidance, that is, from government bodies, in the UK has generally reflected the view that the AIDS epidemic, 'whatever its unique features and however menacing it might appear, is a disease like any other as far as research and treatment is concerned' (cited in Bennett and Ferlie, 1994, p. 62; see, also, advice to employers such as the Department of Employment and Health and Safety Executive's *AIDS and the Workplace*).

This liberal policy stance established at the heart of government policy making is seen to be supported by key aspects of an ideology of *professionalism* that is disseminated principally through the outlook and attitudes of those employed in the management and administration of public medical and welfare services. As Bennett and Ferlie describe it, this is an ideology that seems to equate largely with traditional notions of medical ethics, encapsulating a purportedly 'neutral' scientific humanism:

> Thus the ideology of the profession became institutionalized within government departments dealing with health care issues and, when the issue of AIDS first arose, and government became aware of a potential health crisis to which it must respond, it was to this group of public health physicians that ministers and government officials turned for guidance. Hence this professional ideology emphasizing the controlled, non-judgmental, essentially 'scientific' approach, combined with the norms of 'civilized' behaviour held by liberal mandarins,

mediated the response to the epidemic. (ibid, p. 63)

However, it needs to be recognized that although the 'traditional' ideology of professionalism described by Bennett and Ferlie undoubtedly played a key role in establishing the policy response favoured by the liberal elite, it has also been the subject of challenge from inside this professional grouping. In particular, the 1980s have seen the rise to prominence of a movement termed the 'New Public Health' (NPH) that provides a more eclectic and less traditionally medicalized conception of a professional response. According to Armstrong (1993):

> ... the new public health ... necessitates political activity to promote 'environmentally-friendly' policies; it calls for an ecological approach to health; and, for the individual, it requires an extension from concerns with body boundaries or individual psychology to examination of 'lifestyle'. In its new guise of health promotion, public health is now concerned with generating and monitoring 'political awareness' in its widest sense. (Armstrong, 1993, p. 405)

This notion is particularly pertinent in the context of constructive responses to HIV/AIDS since it exposes within the traditional ideology of expert-professionalism an apparent tendency to ignore the role of social inequalities in the origins of medical problems and thus to deal with the symptoms rather than the causes of many forms of illness. This favours the protection of established interests and the status quo rather than challenging the existing power structures that reproduce such inequalities and their resulting ills. Indeed, this was demonstrated in the previous chapter, where we argued that certain aspects of 'official' and professionally endorsed policy geared to regulating health sector employees could be regarded as defensive in orientation. In contrast NPH is, in principle, democratic in operation, working

> through concrete and effective community action in setting priorities, making decisions, planning strategies and implementing them to achieve better health. At the heart of this process is the empowerment of communities, their ownership and control of their own endeavours and destinies. (Altman, 1994, p. 17)

Applied to HIV/AIDS, the intention is to move away from expert discourses that define the person with AIDS as 'other', the subject of scrutiny, control or assimilation, and replace these with a practice that involves those affected in setting the agenda both for their own medical treatment and their own role in the community, in contrast to the privileged role of the 'expert' supported by the ideology of traditional professionalism.

This notion of community empowerment is a key focus of the *radical ideology*. In the UK, the development and propagation of a radical position on AIDS has been due largely to the gay community, a development reflecting not only the impact of the epidemic upon its members but also the organizational base of an existing, albeit fragmented, community able to draw upon the experiences and expertise of the USA with its more strongly developed tradition of gay/civil rights activism, and its earlier experience of the epidemic. Bennett and Ferlie (op cit) thus suggest that, in addition to the provision of care and services for people affected by HIV/AIDS, the stance of the gay community was to use HIV/AIDS as a platform to promote gay rights (1994, p. 64). As will be discussed below, this can involve pressing for AIDS to be recognized as a workplace issue that exposes the homophobic prejudices held within many organizations and, potentially, a restructuring of existing power relations.

However, as Altman (1994, p. 60) makes clear, it is dangerous to assume that a radical ideology is typically held or endorsed by all people with HIV/AIDS, or that it is the only form of action acceptable to the gay community. Although the connection between homophobia and AIDS is a crucial one within many organizations, gay men are not the only group affected, especially outside the western industrial countries, and it is possible to provide at least some protection and support for people with AIDS without comparable measures to guard against discrimination in terms of sexual orientation. Indeed, as will be discussed below, the debate over the relative merits of coupling protection for people with HIV/AIDS to a radical stance on equal opportunities has provided a significant axis of division within the broad constructive approach. Thus, it may be more appropriate to characterize the radical ideology in terms of a general pressure towards rights for disadvantaged groups rather than specifically gay rights, whilst recognizing the crucial role of gay activists in driving this initiative:

... in western liberal democracies, a belief in the importance of the individual asserting his/her rights was central to the rhetoric of emerging PWA groups, which argued for the centrality of positive people in any approach to the epidemic. The founding statement of the American PWA movement ... stressed the importance of PWA involvement in a language which draws heavily on both the principles of gay and women's liberation and on ideas of patient empowerment. (Altman, 1994, p. 59)

Thus, while these three ideological approaches can be seen as standing in opposition to the defensive orientation outlined in the previous chapter, they each point to significantly different objectives for AIDS related policy. On the one hand, the liberal and traditional professional perspectives (hereafter LTP) imply an 'integration' of AIDS within existing frameworks for dealing with organizational crises, thereby neutralizing its potential as a source of irrational fear and panic. The NPH and radical ideologies (hereafter NPHR), on the other hand, are concerned with confronting and, ultimately, transforming the social prejudices and inequalities that AIDS exposes. In particular, these differences are reflected in the priority which each perspective places on the role of equal opportunities in relation to AIDS. Thus, in LTP thinking AIDS is an issue to be dealt with primarily through occupational health and welfare policy or, in the case of discriminatory action, through existing employment legislation. As such, the main relevance of equal opportunities is in ensuring that discrimination does not take place irrationally against people with HIV/AIDS, a stance that usually involves educational initiatives geared towards the 'normalization' of AIDS and based around medical 'facts and fallacies' (see, below).

Such an approach is also endorsed within a NPHR perspective, but these measures are regarded as necessary rather than sufficient conditions for dealing with AIDS-related issues. Here the equal opportunities dimension of AIDS is viewed widely, as focusing not only upon the medical condition but also on the wider prejudices that give rise to the fear of AIDS. This involves making direct challenges to racism, homophobia, sexism and class prejudice (the latter usually perceived as at the root of drug misuse, see Plant and Plant, 1992), all of which are regarded as integral factors in the matrix of meanings through which AIDS is defined (Small, 1993). Thus, from this perspective it is deemed necessary for an organization to commit itself actively to the fight against AIDS and AIDS-related prejudice: HIV/AIDS becomes part of a 'long agenda' for equal opportunities (Cockburn, 1989; 1991).

In practice, the extent to which this aspect of the long agenda can be established will depend on a number of factors, including the existing equal opportunities culture, the presence of ideologically committed personnel in positions to influence policy decisions, the force of conservative opposition, and the extent to which external pressure groups can bring their influence to bear on organization decision makers. Thus, given these contingencies, in most cases the placing of HIV/AIDS on the long agenda is not automatic but likely to be a subject of challenge and compromise, as will be seen below. Before turning to an exploration of the implications of the long and short agendas within the constructive approach, however, it is first necessary to outline those aspects which are common to each. This is most clearly shown through an analysis of written policy based on the approach adopted in the previous chapter.

Written HIV/AIDS Policy

As will be discussed more fully in chapters 6 and 7, people with HIV/ AIDS are given no specific protection in UK/European employment law and, in this respect, those concerned with preventing discrimination have concentrated their efforts on persuading employers to develop policy responses to the issue. Chapter 2 has already shown that not all policies are necessarily wholly positive towards people affected by HIV/AIDS (often despite assertions to the contrary) and can be highly conditional. Constructive policies, therefore, are those where attempts have been made to minimize or eliminate this element of conditionality. The key differences between defensive and constructive policy are summarized in Table 1.1.

In many key respects, therefore, policy based on constructive principles exhibits a significantly different emphasis from the defensive approach. Again this can be illustrated by reference to UK policies we have examined. Consider first the unconditional statements about the treatment of employees with HIV/AIDS:

> There will be no discrimination in recruitment against applicants on the grounds that the applicant has HIV or AIDS. Applicants will not be refused an offer of work because they have AIDS *or* are anti-body positive.

Table 1.1

Orientation towards people with HIV/AIDS	Defensive policy	Constructive policy
Language	Conditional; Emphasis on 'threat' and 'protection'; Victim-centred and disempowering.	Unconditional; Emphasis on positive image; Empowering.
Procedure	Exclusionary; Surveillance; Control.	Non-exclusionary; System support.
Authority	Primacy of managerial prerogative.	Emphasis on consultation; Consent required for most decisions.
Training/education	Information-giving model	Information-giving plus community-oriented approaches.
Cooperation with extra-organizational bodies	Minimal, perhaps trade unions informed but not involved at early stages.	Early involvement of community based organizations and trade unions.

Applicants who are deemed to be medically fit at the time of recruitment will not be refused an offer of work because they have AIDS *or* HIV infection. Medical fitness will be determined through the usual process of consideration by the Organization's medical advisers.

Likewise regarding exclusion, this policy stance makes disclosure of HIV status a matter for individual decision and emphasizes the need to avoid unilateral management decisions regarding redeployment, this usually being conditional only upon ability to do the job on medical grounds, placing a heavy emphasis on mutual decision-making and respect for individual wishes:

> The Organization has no right to require an individual to disclose that he or she has AIDS or to submit to medical tests for the virus.

> If it becomes known that an employee has AIDS the organization will ensure that resources are available to provide adequate support and any reasonable arrangements to enable work to be continued, on the grounds that to continue working may enable the person to maintain confidence and social contact and fight AIDS with more dignity.

Thus, where differentiation is necessary on medical grounds, care is taken that this is handled in a way which does not result in unfavourable treatment and minimizes the risk of stigmatization. The emphasis is on treating HIV/AIDS as an issue which, in one way or another, involves all employees, requiring positive procedures aimed at encouraging mutual responsibility and support. Indeed, most constructive policies acknowledge explicitly the assistance of trade unions and/or AIDS support organizations in their construction and implementation.

The broad thrust of the constructive approach to policy is captured in the recommendations made by the National AIDS Trust's 'Companies Act!' for an 'equitable AIDS policy' and includes the following:

> The policy must address both HIV and AIDS separately, and the company's response to each should acknowledge they are separate conditions.
> HIV and AIDS can be integrated into existing policies, such as those concerning equal opportunities, sickness leave, etc.

> In an integrated policy, mention must be made of HIV and AIDS, to ensure that staff can obtain the information they need on company practice without having to ask specific questions.

> Any policy must clearly state that discrimination, in any aspect of company activity, against anyone who is HIV positive or who has AIDS will not be tolerated.

The policy should state clearly that AIDS will be treated in the same manner as any other progressive or debilitating illness.

The policy must contain a clear statement on confidentiality, explaining the way in which confidential information will be treated.

The policy must make clear, by outlining or referring to discipline and grievance procedures, what action will be taken if staff breach the terms laid down.

The best model policy will cover areas such as opportunities for redeployment, retraining, flexible working, compassionate leave etc. Where possible these should apply not only to those infected with HIV but also to carers. (National AIDS Trust, 1992, appendix)

Normalization, Medicalization and the Short Agenda

Thus, many constructive policies show a strong tendency towards the normalization of AIDS, that is, to treat it as 'just another disease'. This is considered to reflect an objective assessment of the condition and, simultaneously, to contribute towards the defusing of misinformed social prejudice directed towards people with HIV/AIDS, for example, homophobic attack. This has been especially true of 'integrated policies', for example, those of Marks and Spencer and IBM, as cited by Keay and Leach:

Caring for people is very much part of [Marks and Spencer's] ... philosophy. There is no special policy on HIV/AIDS as the company chooses to treat it in the same way as any other life-threatening medical problem, and guidelines on these are given to all the company's personnel management.

IBM UK provides a health programme tuned to the needs of all employees. AIDS is treated as any other serious illness with complete confidentiality and support. Whatever help is necessary is given to enable employees to continue in work as long as possible. (Keay and Leach, 1993, p. 83)

Certainly the theory of Normalization (or 'ordinary life') has become influential in the field of social care and disability service provision and now appears to be spreading into areas of equal opportunities thinking, especially through the notion of 'diversity management' (Greenslade, 1991; Kandola and Fullerton, 1994a, 1994b). In its influential American version, normalization is understood as the 'creation, support, and defence of valued social roles for people who are at risk of devaluation' (Wolfensberger, 1983, p. 234), the emphasis being on the integration of the devalued person into 'normal' society, including full access to civil rights, and a positive self image. Much of the work in this area has been aimed at people with mental and physical disabilities, although it has also been applied (with reservations, see, below) to racism (Ferns, 1992). From this perspective, policies that seek to separate devalued people, even if benign in intent, are suspect as they set such people apart and thereby create the conditions for an accentuation of difference and its labelling as deviant or stigmatizing. According to Wolfensberger (1972) such labels, or 'role expectations', can have a profound effect upon behaviour and can induce the labelled person to live up — or down [*sic*] — to the expected role characteristics. There are, he suggests, eight general roles that are commonly applied to disadvantaged groups: 'sub-human organism, menace, unspeakable object of dread, object of pity, holy innocent, diseased organism, object of ridicule, eternal child' (Emerson, 1992, p. 6). It is striking, of course, that virtually all of these labels have been applied to people with AIDS (see, for example, Lupton, 1994a) and, in this respect, it would seem that if insights from normalization theory can reduce this tendency then they are to be welcomed. Hence, organizational responses influenced by this approach generally attempt either to incorporate AIDS into existing policies such as health and welfare or, if a separate policy is adopted, to emphasize the essentially medical and objective nature of the condition (HSW, 1990, p. 15). Thus, the intention behind such medicalized/integrated policy is to avoid raising unnecessary fears among organization members, and to create the conditions for people affected to be treated like any other sick employee.

The logic of normalization is often apparent in new developments in the area of equal opportunities which currently go under the label of 'diversity management'. According to two UK exponents of this approach:

The basic concept of managing diversity accepts that the workforce consists of a diverse population of people. The diversity consists of visible and non-visible differences which will include factors such as sex, age, background, race, disability, personality, workstyle. It is founded on the premise that harnessing these differences will create a positive environment in which everybody feels valued, where their talents are being fully utilized and in which organizational goals are met. (Kandola and Fullerton, 1994a, p. 47)

What these writers see as differentiating diversity management from 'traditional' approaches to equal opportunities is the former's uncompromising focus on the individual as the object of policy rather than the group. Certainly, there is within diversity management approaches a strong suspicion of anything that smacks of 'collectivism' or group interests (sometimes in a manner reminiscent of Margaret Thatcher's Hayekian dream that there is 'no such thing as society') on the grounds that it is, firstly, inherently unfair and, secondly, potentially stigmatizing. Regarding fairness, the argument focuses on the assertion that, as not all members of any given group will be similarly disadvantaged, and as members of other collectivities may share a particular disadvantage, it is unfair to target remedial measures on a single group. Diversity management suggests that remedial measures should be needs-driven: that is, available to *all* individuals with a deficiency rather than targeted at specific groups, such as women or ethnic minorities.

The potential for unintended stigmatization is similarly perceived to be a function of the identification of particular groups and their receipt of 'preferential treatment'. This has the effect of bringing what may have been a previously unnoticed disadvantage into public view but, simultaneously creating the impression that any collective remedy is due to 'unfair patronage' rather than ability, thus fuelling jealousy and suspicion. This approach is thus akin to normalization techniques to the extent that it attempts a reconstruction of diversity in line with a standard of normality compatible with organizational objectives — 'ordinary organizational life' — that is defined not by the disadvantaged or 'diverse' but by those who control 'normal' society. In this respect it comes much closer to notions of 'assimilation' than many of its exponents would care to admit.

However, it should be clear that the attempt to establish the asocial, that is, objectively medical, and individualized nature of HIV/AIDS through, for example, its integration within an existing organization policy such as occupational health, is a formal exercise that may reflect little of the lived reality of those affected. Thus, while such a position has much to recommend it, especially in its attempt to remove stigmatizing labels from the condition, it can also encourage a marginalization of identities that are stereotypically associated with AIDS — but which, of course, are also causally independent of it.

In fact, the logic of normalization can carry with it a strong sense of normative prescription. In its early stages of development the theory explicitly prescribed a socially acceptable 'normal' lifestyle (which excluded homosexuality, for example, Nirje, 1980), a stance that, whilst now 'watered down' is still apparent in an uneasy and sometimes suspicious tolerance of 'alternative' lifestyles (see, for example, Wolfensberger and Tullman 1989, p. 218). Indeed, the conservatism implicit in some strands of normalization theory advocates that within any disadvantaged group there should be moves to reduce individual stigmata within the group, reduce the number of deviant [*sic*] people within the group, and 'compensate for' the stigmata or deviances by the addition of 'positively valued manifestations' (Wolfensberger and Thomas 1983, p. 26). Thus, as Ferns (op cit) argues in relation to racism, this conservatism can be abused if it results in the imposition of the cultural norms of the white majority on to the minority Black population: 'If the [conservative] Theme were based on values of race equality, there would be no need to reduce differentness in cultural terms as the cultural variety of people would be valued and the Theme could not be used by people to collude with racism' (Ferns, 1992, p. 143). This can also be a potential difficulty with diversity management approaches, for whilst they claim to respect individual difference, this often appears as highly conditional to the extent that difference is only defined as 'acceptable' if it is capable of contributing to the organization's objectives. Ultimately it is, in effect, diversity on management's terms and, as such, disempowering rather than empowering.

Within the context of strongly normalized HIV/AIDS policy there is, thus, the risk that the concern to define AIDS as an 'ordinary' illness and those with it as 'normal' people will, simultaneously, deny the legitimacy, and suppress the recognition of identities that fall outside this narrow and monocultural conception of normality. By a somewhat perverse irony, therefore, the normalization of AIDS may result in a position whereby the protection of people with HIV/AIDS serves as an excuse or justification for shortening the equal opportunities agenda regarding sexual orientation and anti-racism, on the grounds that drawing attention to these sensitive issues will merely heighten AIDS-prejudice 'by association'. This, of course, fits with Wolfensberger and Thomas's (1983) 'conservatism corollary' principle of normalization (mentioned above) which points to the desirability of reducing the number or variety of 'deviances' or stigmata within a given setting so that 'compensation' can be concentrated on one area of 'abnormality'.

Such a stance may, then, result in a marginalization of the experiences, contributions and needs of those communities most affected by HIV/AIDS, replaced by 'objective' expertise and management (Patton, 1990). This is a particular issue for diversity management approaches since the insistent location of disadvantage as an individual problem to be resolved in a manner contributing to organizational objectives, weakens the legitimacy of critical or alternative perspectives originating in groups seeking to represent collective interests that are supra-organizational. There is a suspicion on the part of many managers, especially in the private sector, of any movement that imports into the organization demands that claim allegiance to principles not amenable to managerial authority and control (Cockburn, 1991; Collinson *et al* 1990). This limits the possibilities of developing organizational strategies that allow disadvantaged individuals to draw strength and support from membership of 'elective communities', that is, 'owning and acknowledging what it is one has in common with the other members, to respect and value oneself alongside others who are like oneself' (Brown and Smith 1992, p. 156). In the case of HIV/AIDS, it ignores the stubborn fact that without the work of community-based organizations and pressure groups, the whole course of the epidemic would have run a very different and almost certainly more repressive course (Altman, 1994). The fact that protection and care for people with HIV/AIDS — and most other disadvantaged groups — has had everywhere to be fought for does little to instil support for the naive faith which diversity management places in the expectation that managers of organizations will arrive at such benign responses spontaneously. Indeed, the very attraction of normalization and integration may be that they remove the perceived danger of having to consider responses to HIV/AIDS that raise the need to confront homophobia and equal opportunities based on sexual orientation as issues in their own right, a dilemma outlined by Cockburn (1991) as characteristic of one of her case-study firms:

> There were men in High Street retail who said without compunction that ... they frankly did not want to share a workplace with 'queers'. In such a climate of opinion it is not surprising that top management and personnel managers were alarmed by their responsibilities concerning AIDS ... How best to defend the employment rights of AIDS sufferers [*sic*], yet avoid an outbreak of hysterical homophobia? (Cockburn 1991, p. 193)

In this respect, there is a potentially serious contradiction between the benefits of normalization that do stem from the uncoupling of a putative causal relationship between sexuality/ethnicity and AIDS and the limitations of an approach that, in return for such a concession, demands that autonomous identities remain largely silent and unacknowledged within 'normal' organizational processes.

Normalized and individualized approaches, however, also raise issues of a more directly practical kind. There is, for instance, the question of whether an organization has in place measures that can deal with discrimination against people with, or suspected of having, HIV/AIDS should this arise. On the one hand, this eventuality may not be covered by many occupational health policies, given that few other illnesses are the basis for comparable prejudicial behaviour. And, on the other hand, a considerable amount of the prejudice evoked by AIDS *is* focused upon social identities rather than upon illness *per se* (see, chapter 4). In this respect, the mere fact that a policy does not draw attention to, or differentiate, AIDS as an 'abnormal' condition does not of itself mean that it will prevent discriminatory attitudes and behaviours. Indeed, one of the reasons frequently cited for developing an equal opportunities oriented response is that it makes explicit the fact that such discrimination will not be tolerated, with a clarity that cannot be achieved by a normalized/medicalized policy. Similarly, the use of diversity management techniques places a heavy emphasis on the voluntary awareness, tolerance and understanding of managers and employees to respond positively to such issues; whether this can ever be fully achieved without the availability of explicit proscription remains an open question.

It can be suggested, therefore, that the crucial issue with a normalizing approach is the extent to which it is supported by other organizational policies that are capable of protecting the interests and identities of those communities that have been most directly affected by the epidemic, but offering this protection *in its own right* rather than as a consequence of contracting a particular illness. Thus, normalization as a means of integration may ignore such protection, or even be used as a reason for not needing to provide it. Indeed, looked at in this light, there may be some difficulties with the view that, of itself, short agenda/normalization approaches can serve as a wholly adequate means of pre-empting homophobic, racist or sexist attack.

In the UK at the present time it must be recognized that many of the documented workplace problems associated with AIDS (and also the anecdotal ones) are concerned directly or indirectly with issues of social prejudice, especially sexuality (see, chapter 5 below). Thus, the normalization of HIV infection can mean that, where an organization has no recognition or protection of the rights and entitlements of, say, lesbians and gay men within its other personnel policies and practices, the potential benefits of an HIV/AIDS policy may be undermined. The case of gay men can be used to illustrate this point. Firstly, regarding the anti-discriminatory aspects of AIDS policy it may be necessary for an organization independently to recognize sexual identity as a basis for prejudicial behaviour to avoid situations where an organization member can claim that they are not discriminating on the basis of AIDS or HIV, whilst doing so on the grounds of sexual orientation.

Secondly, self-disclosure of antibody status is often encouraged by constructive approaches by guaranteeing the certainty that an infected person's employment prospects will be protected and their confidentiality secured. This is intended to allow the medical needs of the person to be met effectively within the context of a job that makes appropriate demands on their physical condition at any given time. However, without wider protection of rights this runs the risk of making disclosure problematic for those who feel that their illness will be linked to some other factor — homosexuality or drug abuse — that they fear will not receive such sympathetic treatment.

Finally, illness and death raise the need for organizations to recognize the responsibilities and commitments of carers not in 'conventional' relationships towards their (ill) partners or dependents, and their right to compassionate/bereavement leave. At present, many organizations, if they provide such benefits at all, operate with a narrow and traditional (that is, heterosexual and male dominated) view of 'family' and 'close relative' and may effectively deny such opportunities to single parents and homosexual couples. Certainly, a measure of hostility to such 'concessions' can be gained from the BBC's decision in 1994 to withdraw one-off wedding gifts to all staff after prominent Conservative MPs complained that such benefits were also extended to same sex couples. The row came to light as the result of an engineer being refused marriage leave by his manager after having taken a 'confirmation of love' vow with his male partner. The Tory MP, Sir Nicholas Fairbairn, commented on BBC Radio that licence payers' money should not be used 'to pay buggers and lesbians to indulge in their perversions on holiday'.

Thus, where an organization is uneasy about the issue of sexual orientation there may also be a tendency for an HIV/AIDS policy, whilst accepted in theory, to be neutralized in practice. Because addressing these issues progressively involves a change in structural aspects of organization and, therefore, power, normalization can appear an attractive option as it focuses on redefining individual opportunities and expectations to meet established organizational practice, rather than vice versa.

Thus, a final problem with the normalization approach is that even if it is successful in defining those with HIV/AIDS as 'merely sick', they are then consigned either to a social group that suffers similar levels of discrimination and prejudice and an absence of civil and employment rights, namely, the disabled (see, for example, Shearer, 1981; Morris, 1993), or dealt with according to the frequently limited and highly variable provision of sickness benefit. The former position is problematic in a number of ways. Firstly, it does not deal comfortably with those people who are HIV positive but asymptomatic and are neither ill nor disabled (except in the sense used by the Americans with Disabilities Act of being limited in one of 'life's major functions', see, chapter 7 below). Secondly, it fails adequately to distinguish between intermittent illness, long-term illness and disability. It needs to be recognized that not all illness is disabling and that to be disabled is not necessarily to be ill or to have a health problem (LAGER, 1992).

In effect, therefore, attempts to normalize and individualize constructive responses to HIV/AIDS, because of their limited challenges to existing patterns of organizational authority, are highly compatible with a 'short agenda' orientation towards equal opportunities whereby new measures are adopted to 'minimize bias in procedures such as recruitment and promotion. It is formal and managerial, but nonetheless desirable' (Cockburn, 1991, p. 218). Thus, a short agenda approach to HIV/AIDS, can deal with the most obvious problems surrounding employment, but the solutions offered may, in practice, be more panacea than remedy. It is this that the NPHR approach seeks to address through a longer agenda for HIV/AIDS.

Challenge, Diversity and the Long Agenda

These difficulties and contradictions have been recognized by many activists in the field who have attempted to resolve them by lengthening the HIV/AIDS dimension of the equal opportunities agenda. In the wake of AIDS panic in the mid-1980s, and in the expectation of a rapid growth in the level of infection, many AIDS pressure groups sought to promote a campaigning and radical style of equal opportunities initiative through which organizations were exhorted publicly to join the fight against AIDS, the latter defined as a social rather than exclusively medical phenomenon. This type of approach seeks to establish what Cockburn (1991) has termed a 'long agenda' for equal opportunities. At its most ambitious this represents a 'project of transformation' for organizations, through which the power of some groups over others is exposed and processes inaugurated to change the nature of that power so as to increase the control ordinary people of diverse kinds have over institutions and to encourage a 'melting away of the white male monoculture' (1991, p. 218). The 'model guidelines' developed by the Lesbian and Gay Employment Rights Group (LAGER) provide an example of this stance in the area of HIV/AIDS:

> This organization is committed to fighting HIV and AIDS related discrimination in all its forms. We will actively fight discrimination against people with AIDS related illnesses, people who are HIV antibody positive and people often assumed to be affected by HIV/AIDS: particularly gay men, intravenous drug users, people with haemophilia and people from Africa. This organization recognizes that there is no such thing as a 'risk group' in relation to HIV and AIDS, only risk behaviour. (LAGER, 1990, p. 3)

Policies constructed in this vein pay particular attention to the social dimension of AIDS prejudice. For example:

There exists within society a negative and condemnatory response to the infection. This may be explained by society's homophobia and the early known transmission of the infection, in the west, amongst the male, homosexual community and injecting drug users ... carrying the infection remains a potentially stigmatizing and alienating experience ... This policy must be read and implemented in the context of the Equal Opportunities Policy, which is applicable to staff who are HIV positive or who have AIDS. These staff are potentially subject to prejudice and disadvantage and, therefore, Equal Opportunities Policy applies to them.

In assessing the needs of, and working with, people who are HIV positive or who have AIDS, the context of the person's race, culture, religious and spiritual belief and sexual orientation must be taken into account.

To promote positive images of, and for people with HIV and with AIDS and to diminish the effects of stigmatization associated with infection. (HIV/AIDS policy, national charity)

This stance has also come to be a concern of most trade unions, albeit after an initially ambivalent response to the epidemic. In an early contribution on this subject Robertson (1987) made a distinction between the responses of two unions, NALGO (National and Local Government Officers Association) and NUPE (National Union of Public Employees), focusing on the tolerance of difference issue discussed above. According to Robertson, NUPE concentrated its attention on demanding action on AIDS from central government, followed by concerns about health and safety, and finally discrimination (1987, p. 148), the reasons for this prioritization lying in this union's wider campaign of opposition to government cuts and the involvement of many of its members in the care of people with AIDS within the health sector. NALGO, in contrast, with its membership primarily in local government, had developed a stronger orientation towards the politics of equal opportunities, not the least of which was a consistent focus on gay and lesbian rights:

... it has encouraged minority groups to organize separately within the union, and has by far the strongest and most active lesbian and gay group of any union. Not surprisingly, therefore, it was from this group of members, who found themselves increasingly under threat in the workplace, that the demand for action first came. The action they demanded was, in the first instance, a campaign aimed at educating and informing the members, and secondly, that the union negotiate protection from employers. (Robertson, 1987, p. 149)

More recently the TGWU (Transport and General Workers Union) policy on HIV/AIDS states, as a key clause, that an important role for the union should be to:

Develop a strategy to protect and extend equal opportunities at work, and in particular, to ensure that all officers actively seek to negotiate equal opportunities policies which include sexual orientation and to prevent discrimination faced by lesbians and gay men and other groups at work. (TGWU, undated)

In these respects the NPHR response seeks to provide a more complete grasp of the contradictions of AIDS than is achieved by normalized/medicalized approaches. In particular, what appears to have emerged from these debates is a strategy to lengthen the AIDS agenda within organizations: seeking a normalization of AIDS in terms of illness is not necessarily undesirable, but it must lead to other initiatives as well. These include striving to promote and protect the integrity of those communities that have been most directly affected by the epidemic, securing civil rights for those who are disabled, a community which many people with HIV/AIDS may eventually join, and developing a positive response to illness.

It is worth reinforcing the point that disability and illness are not necessarily the same thing and need to be addressed as separate policy issues, albeit with an area of overlap. This, in turn, can lead to a call for the restructuring of jobs and working practices to allow those who are sick to have positive access to fulfilling work, rather than merely being protected from arbitrary exclusion. Thus, AIDS itself *can* be downplayed as a 'special issue' but, simultaneously, benefits must be sought for the range of people who will be affected, either directly or indirectly, with a greater emphasis on the empowerment of employees who are ill and/or disabled. However, what is most significant about this approach is the position adopted in relation to the organization of work and employment: it advocates not merely the 'administration' or 'management' of employees with HIV/AIDS according to traditional procedures, but the need for employers to change working practices to accommodate the needs of sick employees. This is quite the reverse of 'normal' managerial solutions in this field, where people with HIV/AIDS, and other illnesses, may be offered incentives — positive or negative — to give up their jobs to avoid the development of 'difficult' situations (see, LAGER, 1992). In essence, then, the NPHR approach offers what may be best termed 'normalization-plus', where the 'plus' refers to a lengthened equal opportunities agenda which formally provides protection for not only people with HIV/AIDS *as such* but also, and independently, for those social groups that have suffered discrimination by association, and for disadvantaged/minority groups in general. In this way, normalizing the illness does not have to run the risk of compromising or marginalizing community identities.

Training and Education

Most workplace training and education about HIV/AIDS has been organized along less than radical lines, generally approximating to what have been termed information-giving and behaviour change models. This approach has clear parallels with the 'short agenda' position as it largely avoids engagement with issues that either challenge or lie outside existing patterns of managerial authority and control. It is essentially a didactic method which assumes that individuals will rationally avoid what they have been warned about. In practice this means a do-it-yourself approach which relies on top-down communication from an 'expert' source, often both literally and metaphorically remote.

An example is the Employment Department and Health Education Authority publication *AIDS and the Workplace* which is intended to provide employers with simple, straightforward information emphasizing that HIV does not constitute a threat within the normal workplace context, and outlining legal responsibilities of employers and good employment practice, including the development of an AIDS policy. The booklet is at pains to establish its basis in fact and frames workplace responses in terms of established good practice, amenable to 'normal' planning procedures and not requiring a significantly different approach from any other human resource issue. This approach is also found in another state-sponsored information sheet, *AIDS and Work*, this time aimed at employees, and subtitled 'The facts employees should know'. The basic message of this sheet is that 'working with someone who has HIV or AIDS does not put you at risk'. In both cases the reader is addressed in a manner which is instructional and presents both facts about the disease and appropriate responses as rationally uncontestable ('sensible').

This factual and didactic approach can be contrasted with a booklet produced by North West Thames HIV Project, entitled *HIV Infection and the Workplace*. The most noticeable difference is that this document sets out firstly to engage the reader rather than to instruct him/her. The illustrations are also interestingly different: *AIDS and the Workplace* shows featureless people in formalized settings, including one of a group of managers (?) being instructed by an 'expert', whereas the NW Thames leaflet uses drawings which evoke personality, activity and realistic idiosyncrasy. Thus, rather than purging the material of emotional and human content in favour of 'facts' and 'instructions' the booklet opens with stories of the situations faced at work by people, with names, affected by HIV.

Although apparently less common, some initiatives have aimed at a wider educational remit, best defined as awareness raising. Here the concern has been to develop in those who have not been affected by HIV a sense of understanding, tolerance and empathy towards those who have. Such understanding it is argued, enables non-infected employees to act compassionately and rationally when dealing with people with HIV/AIDS and, simultaneously, creates the conditions in which the latter can more fully exercise their abilities and rights. In this respect it is an approach that moves towards a long agenda of NPHR by promoting the dissemination of information with an empowering intent, seeking to commit people directly to 'the cause'. This has parallels with the approach characterized by Aggleton and Homans (1987) as the 'socially transformatory model' which attempts to enhance health by 'bringing about far reaching social change throughout society', achieved through 'participatory learning and group work around shared experiences to enable the development of a critical awareness of the societal factors affecting health and well-being' (Aggleton, 1989, p. 223). Although there will still be a concern with 'information-providing' techniques, these are supplemented by a broader focus; consider, for example, the content of a seminar run by a private sector organization:

> ... an understanding of epidemics, sexually transmitted diseases, death, dying, grief, drug use, loss, fear, sexuality, homophobia, prejudice, and the politics and economics of AIDS. Often people have negative attitudes about presumed lifestyles and behaviours. (Policy document, private sector company)

The LAGER (1990) guidelines also suggest that training should be used as a vehicle for consciousness-raising beyond the medical/disease model thereby confronting associated prejudices and prescribing a stance of opposition to these:

> Training will be given to staff and management which challenges the misinformation around HIV and AIDS. Such training should also challenge racist and homophobic connotations associated with the origin and transmission of the virus ... Workers will be encouraged to challenge racist and homophobic connotations associated with HIV/AIDS at all times. (LAGER, 1990, p. 3)

A more cautious form of this approach can be seen to lie behind the National AIDS Trust's 'Companies Act!' initiative, a national charter setting out good practice in relation to HIV/AIDS in the workplace, and encouraging corporate signatories actively to support constructive work in the AIDS field:

> They must achieve one of several goals within the first year. They can educate staff, publicize senior management commitment, raise the issue in the business community, financially support the Charter and the Trust, or provide practical help to any HIV/AIDS agency.

There are over 40 signatories to the Charter, including companies such as Marks and Spencer, IBM, and National Westminster Bank. The philosophy of Companies Act! suggests that 'HIV should be on every personnel manager's agenda; a non-discriminatory policy is the only practical approach. HIV and AIDS are equal opportunities issues, not exclusively health and safety ones'. However, even such 'high profile' commitments to the fight against AIDS are not without their practical difficulties, a point that is well made in Robertson's (1987) discussion of trade union policy, which applies equally to other forms of organization:

First, many of the unions which have produced a detailed policy have failed to effectively communicate that policy to its members. Second, it is impossible to judge a union's response in isolation from the structure and membership of that union, and the climate in which the policy was drawn up. Third, looking at its policies alone does not tell us much about how a particular union is likely to respond to individual cases. Many trade unions which have excellent policies on paper have failed to support individual workers, whilst other unions which may perhaps have no official policy on AIDS have proved to be very supportive when approached by their members for assistance. (Robertson, 1987, p. 146)

Conclusions

Although the length of the agendas associated with constructive responses is variable, any such approach faces the major problem of translating policy into practice. First, is the fact that formal policy is a management tool, the nature and objectives of which may or may not be understood or shared by other sections of a workforce. Alternatively, there are situations where the process of policy formation is an end in itself, a demonstration of corporate planners' competence rather than a real exercise in the management of change. Coupled to this is the fact that an organization's management itself is not a homogeneous grouping, and a policy developed by, say, a personnel department or corporate head office, may be regarded as irrelevant and inappropriate by other managers who orientate their actions and attitudes toward more instrumental local objectives (Collinson, 1991). As such, the policy may be ignored or side-lined unless rigorously and continuously enforced through explicit mechanisms of cultural support. This is likely to be a particular problem for long agenda approaches as these generally demand both a commitment to an ideal of transformation and a willingness to initiate significant changes to established management practices and responsibilities. In this sense, it is not only active resistance that may challenge the effective adoption of a policy but also the simple failure of some managers to take it seriously and to convey its message with indifference and apathy, thereby signalling to subordinates its de facto status as an irrelevance to be ignored rather than enforced. Even in organizations with a strong formal commitment to constructive policy, the objectives of a long agenda do not exist in a vacuum, as a personnel manager from one of the companies included in our own research (see, chapter 4 below) explained:

> If you know if somebody has the HIV virus or they actually divulge that, then our policy is that we wouldn't discriminate against that person. Now that's the policy, its never been put to the test so that's very difficult for me to make any comment as to whether that would be allowed to continue. I'm not sure if somebody was to come for a job interview and divulged to the person there that they were HIV positive, I'm not sure whether, even if they were the right candidate for the job, how that would be looked on because its never been put to the test as far as we know ... that is how I would see it because my experience here is that even with disability, that if people have a choice between an able bodied person and a disabled person they will automatically go for an able bodied person because the job has got to be done ... The same would apply if they announced that they were HIV positive, I can't honestly believe that a manager will say, 'Oh yes, I want you'. But its never been proved.

This form of 'instrumental pragmatism' at operational level may also help to explain the fact that there are numerous cases of less favourable treatment being given to people with HIV/AIDS in organizations that have official policies that could be categorized as constructive (LAGER, 1992; Arkin, 1994).

As interest in and concern about the epidemic has waned in both popular and specialist media, so keeping up the pressure for a longer agenda has proved difficult. As the predicted spread of HIV does not seem to have had the dramatic effects predicted in the late 1980s, and in the face of a long and deep recession, attention within many work organizations has focused on more immediate issues. Against these, HIV/AIDS has come to be perceived as a minority issue within most work organizations and, like most other such issues, is allocated scant attention when the interests of the majority are threatened by economic collapse. Even without the impact of recession, however, it is likely that the apparent failure of the epidemic seriously to touch the heterosexual population, and its effective decline as a popular news issue, would, in any event, have made it a low priority issue for most employers, as the following account concerning Barclays Bank (a Companies Act! signatory) illustrates:

> But supporting an AIDS policy with an employee education programme poses its own problems for employers, especially at a time when most training budgets are already stretched. As Christine Lyles, of Barclays Bank asks: 'If you ran a seminar or workshop when the incidence of the illness was very, very low, when would you run it again? Next year? The year after? (Arkin, 1994, p. 35)

The results from our own research suggest that the framing of AIDS as an imminent and dangerous threat to organizations and their employees did not reflect the perceptions of our respondents. But to dismiss it as an irrelevance or an issue of no concern would also be mistaken. Concerns about AIDS have not disappeared, but now seem to rest at a deeper level of understanding, one which relates to practical and specific actions, and where there remains an underlying uncertainty and apprehension. Thus, should AIDS dramatically re-enter the public agenda, or should individual workplaces have to deal with cases of HIV/AIDS, it is still likely to cause difficulty — even in many organizations that have adopted a formally constructive response. Indeed, we see little clear evidence that the current ambivalence and lack of concern could not be easily translated into renewed discriminatory action and, in this respect, the need remains to continue working for a longer agenda that can pursue not only AIDS but also the related inequalities and injustices that surround it. It is to a discussion of these underlying concerns and their organizational ramifications that the following chapters are devoted.

Chapter 4

HIV/AIDS and Workplace Dilemmas

Introduction

In most organizations, formal responses to AIDS are devised by functional specialists such as personnel or occupational health managers, usually in response to the prompting of government agencies, professional bodies, media attention and, perhaps, direct experience. Such responses generally reflect the particular concerns identified by these managers as relevant to the organization and are then amended, either by addition or deletion, through a process of scrutiny by senior management or a management dominated committee system. While this may subject the issue of AIDS to considerable discussion and the expression of divergent interests, it remains a process in which most of the participants are, usually by the very fact of their involvement and consequent access to relevant information, relatively well informed. In addition, they also bring to the discussion certain formal role expectations, that is, as managers charged with ensuring organizational efficiency, or as representatives of a given constituency such as a department or trade union.

However, for those organization members not involved in such a policy-making process their interest in and understandings of HIV/AIDS may be very different. Thus, where the views of policy makers are neither shared nor understood this can result in overt or covert resistance to policy goals, or simply their neglect. In the former case, resistance may be directed against policies that are seen to be too tolerant of people with HIV/AIDS or, conversely, those that are perceived to be too repressive. In the latter case, that is, of neglect, which is probably more common, the policy may be regarded as irrelevant, with organization members perhaps unaware of its existence. Thus, as can also happen in organizations where no formal policy has been developed, members respond to HIV/AIDS by drawing upon normative frameworks that have been developed either outside the organization or through informal work-group interaction.

In this respect, it is not sufficient to examine only managerial definitions or to take the formal articulation of organization policy as an accurate guide to actual behaviour. The representation of an issue as formal policy is never wholly complete: it is, by definition, a simplification, an abstraction from a 'messy' reality. Thus although the intention is to make a situation or phenomenon 'knowable', the abstract packaging of the issue may be too insensitive to provide guidance in specific situations. Indeed, because of the nature of the media attention it has attracted, HIV/AIDS engages most people at a subjective level: not only is it widely perceived as a threat to human-kind, but it also taps deeply rooted ideas about identity, propriety and mortality, often with associations of 'good' and 'evil':

> Sexuality, social marginality and disease intersect in a matrix that is, itself, both an indicator of the social anxiety and a conductor of the social tension that are central to both personal identity and social policy. AIDS has become the symbolic bearer to a host of meanings about contemporary culture — its social composition, racial boundaries, attitudes to social marginality, moral configurations and social mores ... (Small, 1993, p. 90)

This matrix of meanings which surrounds HIV/AIDS connects not only with the pragmatic concerns of the formal responses outlined in the previous chapters, but also with the emotions and feelings of organization members which, according to Fineman (1993, p. 15), provide the 'social glue' that 'will make or break organizational structures and gatherings' — including those relating to HIV/AIDS.

Emotion, Organization and HIV/AIDS

There has been a growing interest in the role of emotion in organiza-tions and a recognition that the existence of formal and bureaucratic procedures, while they may proscribe them, do not prevent emotional involvements and responses. However, emotions do not exist in some 'essential' or fundamentally irreducible sense, but are, at least in significant part, socially constructed, framed by reference to established standards of behaviour and by personal experience — both direct and vicarious (Ashforth and Humphrey, 1993; Fineman, op cit, ch.1).

For people with HIV/AIDS, for example, there may be anger and resentment in the face of blatant discrimination, as one ex-dancer explains:

> ... the theatre [revolves around looks]; if I told anyone in the business I had AIDS I'd never work again. Last year I had to give up my job ... The theatre does a lot for AIDS in terms of charity events and so on but secretly, under the surface, there is a financial consideration which is that they don't want to employ somebody who is a liability. Now I've cut out a lot of my theatre friends. I think it would give some of them great pleasure to know that I'm lying in a hospital bed. (Veksner and Lane, 1993, p. 18)

For many, though, these feelings are also tinged with a complex mix of other emotions. Using a series of in-depth interviews with 66 people with HIV and a matched control sample, Green (1995) provides insights into the experience of gaining and keeping employment in the face of a positive HIV diagnosis. What emerges clearly from the accounts provided by Green is the combined effect upon the individual of the physical and psychological effect of HIV infection on the one hand, and the demands and responsibilities of employment on the other. Thus, although a number of her respondents gave up their jobs because they became too ill, others stopped working because they felt the demands of their job would, ultimately, have a detrimental effect on their health, or because their psychological state was so disturbed by the HIV diagnosis that they felt unable to perform their work effectively. In addition, six of Green's respondents reported overt discrimination as a result of their HIV status, thus:

> 1. A haemophiliac went for two interviews and reported that the atmosphere changed immediately after he mentioned HIV and he was not offered either job ...
> 2. An engineer working on short-term contract in the Third World was unable to keep his diagnosis confidential. His employers refused to renew his contract when it expired,

although previous renewals of contract had been straight-forward.

3. A young teacher who had informed his employer of his HIV status failed to be promoted although he felt he was the most qualified applicant for the job.

4. An army wife reported that her husband's career was ruined following her diagnosis, although he tested HIV-negative. He was confined to working in a restricted number of countries and his opportunities for advancement were severely restricted ...

5. A health professional was told by his European employers to leave after being diagnosed with HIV, as the country he was working in did not permit HIV-positive foreigners to reside there.

6. A sex worker was sacked when her colleagues found out she was HIV-positive and refused to work with her. (Green, 1995, p. 257–8)

Running through these accounts are the themes of guilt, fear and insecurity: fear that employers or colleagues will find out about their HIV status and respond negatively, and guilt about 'having to live a lie' by concealing their status or fearing that they would put others at risk. These are illustrated by the following quotations from Green's interviews, the first with a chef and the second a trainee creche worker:

I would be very nervous of starting again. As a chef I had great flair for knife control ... I'm very fast with a blade and sometimes you just nick yourself and because the blade's that sharp you don't notice until half the food is ruined. You can't walk into a restaurant, cut your finger and throw the whole tray out or say I cannae work tonight, I've got a wee scratch on my finger. Most chefs would just put a plaster on and get on with it. With me I'd have to stop work.

Well ... as far as my supervisor is concerned I am fit. But it's just that for some reason if it got out that I was HIV positive, well you can imagine how parents would feel. You know they'd be terrified and I can understand ... So he's got to see various people about that before he actually signs the forms to keep

> himself in the right and also to keep me in the right ... I wouldn't want him to put himself in jeopardy. (Green, 1995, p. 258)

This emotional mix is repeated in many of the US cases examined by Cameron (1993), for example:

> 'Before quitting my job,' she [Lisa, a computer programmer] said, 'I didn't know if I should. I'd be sick and then I'd be better. *They needed to count on me. They have the right to that. They knew about the AIDS and were supportive.*' 'There were good reasons for me to stay in my job,' Lisa continued. 'I liked having the money. It provided me with insurance. Staying at work provided me with something to do and a good way of self-esteem. There were good reasons to quit my job. It was healthier for me not to be working because it was putting a great deal of strain on me. Now that I've quit my job there are good reasons to go back to work. My health insurance ends in 2 years. I'm bored.' (Cameron, 1993, pp. 105–6)

In addition, Green (op cit) makes use of the notions of 'enacted stigma' (active discrimination) and 'felt stigma' (fear of discrimination) to explore people with AIDS' self-perception of their condition compared to that of the 'general public'. She suggests that although, in practice, felt stigma may be more prevalent than enacted stigma, the former is nonetheless damaging in its effects upon the self-image and actions of the person concerned. This is especially the case in relation to employment, as the *expectation* of others' adverse reactions seems as powerful as *actual* discrimination in dissuading a person with HIV from seeking or keeping a job. While such a reaction may be, in part, an internal psychological response to the trauma of diagnosis, it also has organizational ramifications in terms of emotion management and emotional display rules, in particular, the extent to which other organization members feel able or willing to accept the 'emotional labour' involved in working with someone who is known to be HIV positive. Such 'acceptance' however, is unlikely to be simply a matter of individual volition, for as Ashforth and Humphrey (1993) point out, there may be numerous constraints placed upon the articulation of emotion within organizations. They point to the pejorative view of emotion that operates within most organizations and identify a number of mechanisms through which the 'socially acceptable' expression of emotion is regulated, including those of neutralizing, normalizing and prescribing.

Neutralizing techniques involve the development of organizational processes and procedures designed to contain a potentially emotional experience within a purportedly rational framework, thereby minimising its potentially disruptive effects. This appears to be one function of HIV/AIDS policies which, in various ways, seek to make the 'management' of HIV/AIDS predictable and amenable to organizational control (Goss, 1994a).

Normalizing tactics are intended to deal with those emotional expressions that cannot or have not been neutralized by deploying a process of reframing whereby emotional feelings are concealed beneath explanations couched in apparently rational terms, for example, by defining HIV/AIDS as a strictly occupational health issue as a means of avoiding the need to confront emotionally loaded feelings which surround sexual and racial identity and drug use.

Prescription attempts to define 'acceptable' emotional expressions within the context of organizational activity. Thus, emotion is seen not as an uncontrollable outburst of feeling but as something to be 'managed' in a manner constrained by the exigencies of organizational need. In relation to HIV/AIDS this has been a particular concern in the field of health care where professional bodies have felt it necessary to establish appropriate emotional responses, proscribing expressions of fear, hate or disapproval and prescribing those of courage, care and concern (Sim, 1992, p. 572).

More generally, this form of prescription has been present in almost all ideologies of industrial work which assert the need for 'irrationality' to be restrained, but it has also been subject to conscious manipulation through attempts to use 'managed emotion' as a means of enhancing organizational performance, embodied in many of the attempts of 'human relations' theorists to improve motivation by cultivating forms of sociability through 'open management' and team-based work. Such attempts, however, have always had their limits, expressed in the notion of 'tough love' which gained currency in human resource management thinking in the 1980s:

> The needs of our business will be most effectively attained if the needs of people for fulfilment, success, and meaning, are met.
> If people are in poor shape, the company's objectives are

unlikely to be achieved. Yet the needs of the business still come first. People need to be developed, but this will not be achieved by treating them with 'soft care', by allowing issues to be smoothed over without being properly addressed. To treat people without care will cause them and, therefore the business, to diminish. Experience suggests that the needs of people and the business will be best met if we treat ourselves with 'tough love.' ... People, of course, are far and away the most important resource in any company. But they are not more than that. It is very easy to forget when endeavouring to develop people and to care for them, and even to love them, that the needs of the business must come first. (cited in Legge, 1989, p. 33)

These techniques of emotional regulation demonstrate some of the ways in which emotional expression is socially constructed within organizations, constrained by formal and informal rules and, thus, highly conditional. Given that people with HIV will, as employees, have gained a knowledge of these rules through their previous work experiences, it is perhaps hardly surprising that they anticipate being subject to discrimination and/or stigma. Indeed, if we accept Green's finding (1995, above) that the general public express views that are largely liberal and supportive towards people with HIV/AIDS in the abstract, this does not mean that such principles will be converted into action under specific conditions. As has been suggested, organizations are not environments where people do, or can, act simply in response to their feelings, but where such feelings are cross-cut and constrained by other interests which may be afforded higher priorities. The techniques of emotion management outlined above, for instance, provide mechanisms whereby certain individual feelings, which may be strongly held in private, can be legitimately suspended within the public world of organizational activity.

Such suspension, however, is not necessarily an easy or automatic option, but may be the source of considerable 'soul searching', often presenting individuals with difficult moral choices. Indeed, the tensions involved in sustaining an appropriate emotion management rule-set are described by Sievers (1993) within the context of a charity organization run by positive and non-positive people:

As time passed, the condition of the HIV-infected members who had previously not been ill worsened drastically and some had already died. As a consequence they had to change roles from managers and helpers to ill or even dying patients. . . . Although the institution felt obliged to maintain the employment of the seriously ill, because of limited financial resources it was forced to reduce the help it had intended to provide. Because no-one could seriously suggest dismissing the sick and making them eligible only for reduced unemployment benefits or social security, the non-infected were supposed to reduce their jobs to part-time. But since the institution depended on them, it meant that they were supposed to also work part-time as volunteers. This began a vicious circle. Most of the non-infected were, in addition to their own superhuman commitment, supposed to earn their living through this work. And as they were already earning much less than in comparable jobs, they personally felt disregarded and neglected. Though they were used to not getting any gratitude from the infected (with some exceptions), they now had to cope with envy. They had always been aware of the usually unspoken envy of the infected about their longer life-expectancies; now they felt envious themselves of their former colleagues, who, despite their inability to work, received a higher income leaving them, the uninfected, to cope with the burden of underemployment and increasing demands for help from the outside. (Sievers, 1993)

That emotional responses such as these are focused and sharpened by the organization of work is, to some extent, inescapable as individuals invest more or less of their identity in a job role shaped by and for the technical and economic demands of organizational objectives. This, of course, applies not only to people with HIV/AIDS but also to other organization members.

These types of emotional conflicts are discussed by Banas (1992), for example, in his account of managing subordinates with AIDS. Banas describes how, as a newly appointed administrative director at the US Comptroller of the Currency, he had to respond to two successive cases of junior managers becoming ill with AIDS.

Jim walked into my office . . . sat down stiffly in his chair, and told me quite calmly that he had just learned he was HIV-positive. I had a hard time taking it in, and when I did I was

> more than surprised. I was devastated. Deep inside, I'm sorry to
> say, a selfish voice was saying, 'Why me?' and 'Not again!' Aloud
> I said, 'I'm terribly sorry to hear that Jim. Please let me know
> if there's anything I can do to help' ... My response was
> superficial and inadequate ... Having been through this once
> before, my compassion was mingled with dread. I didn't want to
> watch Jim suffer, and I didn't want to grapple again with the
> problems that his suffering might cause for his staff and for me.
> (Banas, 1992, p. 28)

In the course of our own research we have spoken to several personnel
managers who, after having to deal with an employee with AIDS, felt
considerable guilt and anxiety about the way in which they handled
matters: whether, for example, they were aware of difficulties early
enough, whether they had provided the right kind and level of support,
whether they had handled the issue of confidentiality appropriately, and
how they had subsequently explained and dealt with the feelings of
co-workers following the employee's death. Indeed, these feelings of
grief and guilt were not confined to personnel managers and often
extended to colleagues, particularly when they only learned that AIDS
had been the cause of a co-workers's death after the event, and then
started to consider how they might have responded differently towards
them had they known. Kirp (1989), for instance, provides a US example
that describes one such 'transformation' in almost revelatory terms:

> Chuck Woodman hadn't always been so concerned about
> people with AIDS. To his subordinates Woodman had a
> reputation as a tough guy, a self-described redneck whose
> heroes included John Wayne and George Patton.... Wood-
> man's attitude about AIDS began to change when he was
> transferred to San Francisco. He remembers how he was
> affected by a funeral for a worker who had died of AIDS ... 'As
> I listened to that minister talking about how angry it made him
> that people with AIDS were shunned, I began to feel some of
> that anger', Woodman says.... After the first funeral Woodman
> started asking questions. 'What can we do for the people with
> AIDS on the job?' he wondered. (Kirp, 1989, p. 141)

Other emotional experiences, however, include despair and depres-
sion resulting from work which carries an inherently high emotional

loading, such as caring for people with AIDS and being closely involved in their progressive illness and death. These are likely to be felt most acutely in areas where dealing with death on a regular basis has not been familiar, but where the nature of client care has always been premised on the close involvement of the service provider. In one of the social service departments covered by our study, for instance, workers in a specialist HIV section spoke of the emotional drain they experienced on the death of clients whom they had come to regard as friends. Initially care workers from this department had attended the funerals of all such clients, but many now expressed a sense of guilt at being unable to sustain emotionally such close involvement and adopting an increasingly detached role, one result of which was the formulation of an informal rule that case workers would stop attending client's funerals, except in exceptional cases. Thus, whereas in traditional medical settings, rules for the emotional management of patient suffering and death are well established and institutionalized, usually involving a combination of personal detachment and joking behaviour ('buffering', in the terms used by Ashforth and Humphrey, op cit). It seems likely that the development of comparable rules may be the source of considerable tension and guilt in newer areas of terminal care provision where such a response may be perceived as callous, uncaring and unprofessional.

HIV/AIDS and Workplace Dilemmas

These accounts illustrate the ways in which the emotional colouring of AIDS, as it confronts the principles of organizational rationality, frequently takes the form of a 'dilemma'. The usual features of a dilemma (see, for example, Toffler, 1986) include the following: it is difficult to isolate as a single unambiguous issue involving clear abstract principles, usually because it is heavily embedded in a specific context that makes it seem highly personal and often unique; similarly, it may appear to involve a number of competing values (rather than just right or wrong), and competing stakeholders such that there is no simple resolution readily apparent; and finally, it confronts those involved with choices which they may feel ill-equipped to make because of limited knowledge.

Further illustration of the ways in which HIV/AIDS can generate dilemmas for organization members is provided by our own empirical research. In this study, 11 organizations were investigated, with an average of 10 employee interviews per organization, a total of 106 respondents. Each interview lasted between half-an-hour and two hours, was tape recorded and transcribed in full. Wherever possible interviews in each organization covered senior managers, line managers, clerical and manual workers. The organizations studied were drawn from the manufacturing, health care, voluntary/charity, hospitality, and public sectors and were located across the UK, although predominantly in the south east. The purpose of the material presented below is not to make grand generalizations but, rather, to point to the inherent complexities of meaning and interpretation that surround this issue. There is a persistent theme of uncertainty — in terms of how employers and employees *should* respond to someone with HIV/AIDS, and how it was anticipated they *would* act — which mirrors that found in the responses of people with HIV (especially those interviewed by Green, 1995, above). Thus, for the respondents in our study, although HIV/AIDS was not a cause of immediate concern or panic in relation to work-related activity, most exhibited a 'background concern' rooted in an inadequate understanding of the virus and the exact nature of work-related risk. This uncertainty meant that many respondents felt ill-prepared to deal effectively with issues attributable to HIV infection in workplace settings, and the vast majority felt the need for more and better HIV information and training of a kind directly relevant to workplace situations. This applied in most of the organizations with 'constructive' policies, supporting our earlier caution regarding the partial role of formal policies in ordering and articulating workplaces responses (see, chapter 3 above).

Thus, although explicit concern about infection at work did not loom large among respondents, anxiety about contact with blood was voiced in work situations where injury, especially cuts, were a common occurrence (the manufacturing shopfloors and the hotel and catering establishments). In non-physical work settings where fewer such concerns were raised, there remained worries in the context of first-aid. Few of those who expressed such fear had received any information or training about HIV/AIDS from their employer and most relied upon an often hazy knowledge acquired from public health broadcasts and the media. For example:

> I have been involved in areas where there is likely to be a violent situation and sometimes one has to go in and, should we say,

sort out the problems of violence where someone has been injured. There has been times when the doubts have crept into my mind: should I be wearing gloves, should I be doing this? ... to a certain degree it's on one's mind. (Nightclub manager)

I'll tell you what I have thought about, somebody said to me, 'Wouldn't you like to be a first aider?' and I said, 'No I wouldn't', because I am not very keen on blood, and I don't think I could give resuscitation to anybody who had AIDS. But I mean there's probably ways and means where you wouldn't catch it but I wouldn't know without somebody giving some sort of information on it. (Supervisor, charity)

A small number of respondents, mostly in managerial positions, regarded HIV/AIDS as an issue of wider relevance to workplace activity. In some cases concern had been sparked by first-hand experience of dealing with employees or clients with the virus, while others had received specific training, but in virtually all instances an element of uncertainty remained predominant. The following are illustrative:

I thought it was foolhardy to work on the assumption that it was never going to happen here, by the law of averages, I guess its going to happen in most organizations at some point, and I am also perfectly aware of the fact that if we do get a member of staff with AIDS then the person that they come to, to say, 'What do we do now?' is me. I thought probably I ought to be better aware than I was. (Personnel manager, charity)

Because I am a counsellor and I go through continuous training sessions, and quite often you were talking about HIV and AIDS, and we've had many workshops dealing with HIV and AIDS. And it was from that I used to come back [to work] and say, 'Hey, come on, we've got to be doing something!' Sooner or later somebody is going to knock on the door and say, 'I have a problem which I think you need to know about and how are we going to deal with it?'. (Personnel manager, distribution)

For these relatively well aware respondents, uncertainty focused on the availability of organizational procedures that would allow a response to people with HIV/AIDS that was ethically sound. For most of those we interviewed, however, uncertainty translated into a more individual concern with risk.

Here the parameters of the dilemma appeared as a choice between an often vague notion of possible risk, the responsibility to protect both staff and clients from this, and a concern with the rights of the person with HIV. In most cases, then, the concern with risk was not simply the result of fear for personal safety but a more complex expression of a sense of duty and obligation framed within the specific context of employment. In short, and recalling the views of Banas (1992, above), there was often a constant dilemma between the anxiety of infection and the desire to 'do the right thing', both by the organization and those individuals directly and indirectly affected. Consider the following:

> It depends where I was going to put them at work. Like I said, it's ignorance ... If I thought I could do something then I would want to know. If there was like a leaflet and instructions and I knew that whoever I put them with was never going to catch it then that's fine by me, but if I thought in the situation whereby you could transmit it by cuts and things then I think I would want to know and I probably wouldn't put them in that area anyway. I would put them somewhere, where they were totally on their own, not on their own exactly, but on their own. (Supervisor, charity)

If the discussion of defensive policy in chapter 2 (above) is recalled, it can be seen how the way in which such policy constructs choices that privilege organizational interests might easily sway individuals experiencing this type of dilemma to opt for actions that disadvantage the person with HIV/AIDS.

Returning to the perception of risk, there were a handful of respondents who exhibited a much higher perception of risk and who tended to favour some form of employer regulation to control what they feared to be the likely adverse and unacceptable effects of HIV in the workplace. However, it should also be noted that these responses may represent a 'normalizing' of emotional fears, that is, the reframing of a deeper mistrust about 'outsiders' (for example, homosexuals or drug-users) into organizationally 'rational' objections presumed to be more acceptable than open expressions of 'real' feelings (Ashforth and

Humphrey, op cit). Certainly, those respondents who expressed the highest perception of risk were also those who, at other points in the interviews, exhibited the most hostile responses towards those they perceived as associated with the spread of HIV (see, chapter 5 below). Thus:

I wouldn't like anybody behind the bar to be employed who is HIV positive, if cuts happen, constant contact with liquids that are drunk by customers, coming into contact with customers ... I wouldn't expect them to be handling the glassware ... [Testing] wouldn't be a bad idea, I personally wouldn't give objections if someone tested me ... Yes I would think that would be a pretty good thing actually. Yes, that would be good. (Manager, nightclub)

I mean even in my kind of job you are always cutting yourself on the metal. When you cut yourself you leave blood on the metal and the next person picks it up ... unless I'm ignorant of that part but I think blood is one of the main factors ... They should perhaps find him a job where perhaps you minimise the risk, in a way that you can't catch it. I know it's a sorry state, but that's it. I mean if you have got anything they put you in hospital and keep you away from other people, whatever it is, not only that, any disease, that's contagious, they keep you away. (Metal worker)

When it comes to people dealing with food and say for example, to keep an employee in the kitchen who had AIDS, if she cut her finger and is sort of mixing some dough and some blood was getting into the dough then that person would get AIDS, then she is basically killing someone, isn't she? (Waitress, nightclub)

How can it be transmitted? If it can be transmitted on money, you know things like that ... maybe it can be transmitted through food, maybe it can be transmitted through something else ... obviously we're prone to say cuts and things like that in the kitchen, I'm in contact with raw meat and things like that so there's cross-contamination there. (Chef, public sector)

Here again, however, motives appeared to be mixed, in most cases involving at least some consideration of work-related responsibility. Although there was not widespread support for employer measures to identify people with HIV, either at the point of recruitment via testing or through self-disclosure, support for testing and mandatory disclosure of HIV status often came from respondents who held a high perception of risk and who (also) worked in areas where the chance of injury and spillage of blood was greatest. With the exception of this small group, most respondents' views on testing and disclosure were often ambivalent and highly conditional. The following quotations illustrate the range of opinion (i.e., from outright opposition, through ambivalence, to support):

> Definitely not [testing]. Particularly not medical work because it's obviously going to be used against them. First of all it's damaging to the individual concerned, there are all sorts of reasons to undergo HIV testing but there are all sorts of reasons not to as well. They shouldn't be forced to take one by an employer or an insurance agency whatever. They would have to deal with the upshot of that. Also it could only be used to work against them. If you test positive it isn't exactly going to work in your favour. (Social worker)

> I mean I wouldn't object to it if it was part of the basic contract, but I would have to have a very good answer as to why they wanted it done, but if it was on a medical side and I was going say as a sick berth attendant I would expect it almost as a mandatory question. Mostly because of the close physical contact ... If you were a prospective employer and you knew that the guy, or girl, that you was employing was HIV free, and the nature of the job might be delicate, then it would probably give you more confidence, or choice to employ them. Not that I'm saying you should not employ HIV positive people, it just depends on the context of the job, doesn't it? (Metal worker)

> Maybe we should introduce a medical and incorporate that into it. Yes I guess, my personal opinion is that if somebody is HIV positive, they ought to declare that they are. I think it should be a statutory regulation that people should declare if they are HIV positive ... I don't think we should employ people who are

> HIV positive ... it's a contagious illness/disease whatever you want to call it. It may not be contagious in the same way that the plague is or TB, something like that but it is still contagious so therefore you shouldn't be in contact with the public. (Nightclub supervisor)

However, apart from those respondents who had strong objections to testing and employer surveillance on principle, a clear majority of respondents felt that workers involved in medical fields and close personal contact should be subject to testing, even if they did not see this as appropriate to their own workplaces. For most non-medical organizations, though, the bulk of respondents were in favour of some form of employer protocol for dealing with AIDS-related issues, seeing this as a more realistic and practical solution than either testing or mandatory self-disclosure. But here again, uncertainty and ambivalence were apparent, some respondents wanting formal rules to establish and safeguard the rights of people with HIV, whilst others envisaged rules designed to protect individuals and the organization from them.

When asked about their expected reactions to working with someone known to be HIV positive a range of responses similar to those previously discussed emerged: from a (single) refusal to mix with such a person to a commitment to provide help and support. Very few respondents, however, had knowingly worked with colleagues or clients who were HIV positive and, as such, their responses must be seen in this light, that is, as based on intention rather than experience. Illustrations of these different responses are provided below:

> They wouldn't work here. They would be fired straight away ... there would just be an atmosphere in there all the time ... I would keep away. (Nightclub manager)

> I would be silly to say it wouldn't unnerve me because it would. I wouldn't want to work with someone who is HIV positive. (Nightclub waitress)

> If you know someone's got the potential to giving you a serious illness, it's human nature that there is that threat ... I don't think you can lose that stigma. Once you know that someone has got it, they've got the potential, the disaster, they can give

it to you, even if you only perceive it as a threat. You might not like being in close proximity to them, you'd be quite happy to sit at a desk together but when it comes to physical contact ... (Local authority officer)

Other than a few examples of clearly articulated non-acceptance, there was little in our data to suggest that employees with HIV/AIDS would, a priori and automatically, be the subjects of prejudice and discrimination. At the same time, however, neither was there overwhelming evidence that they would be treated like any other employee with a medical condition, although the latter seemed more likely than the former — at least in intention (and in the organizations we studied).

Certainly, for many respondents their uncertainty on this issue was coupled to a self-confessed lack of understanding of the virus and its implications. It is in this respect that workplace education and training may have an important role to play. As already stated, the issue of training and information was presented by many respondents as the lynch-pin of workplace responses to HIV. Here again, however, there were a variety of ways in which the nature and effectiveness of training were articulated. One pattern to emerge was a rudimentary hierarchical ordering of the type of information that respondents wanted. In general, those who felt themselves to be fundamentally ignorant and/or perceived a high probability of risk were most concerned to receive material focusing on basic practical/medical 'facts' about transmission, located clearly within the context of their work. In contrast, those already equipped with such an understanding were more concerned to have information relating to the human and social implications at work, coupled to regular reviews of medical developments. The potential for disjunction between the 'biological' and the 'social' approaches to training, however, was raised by one respondent (echoing the interpretation made in the previous section). This manager felt that AIDS training should be closely allied to issues of equal opportunities rather than given a purely 'medical' perspective:

I think the general awareness of it is more important. I think the factual stuff is partial but I wouldn't want a course purely on that because then it's in a sense St John's Ambulances and again that just sends you away getting hysterical about distort blood etc ... (Local authority clerk)

This respondent's objection to the 'medical approach' was that it could result in a reversal of the real priorities arising from HIV to the extent that 'medicalization' tended to emphasize risk and threat — which in the workplace are practically insignificant — instead of providing assistance to those likely to be affected by the disease. It was certainly the case that the training sessions that were most easily recalled and which had made the deepest impact on respondents were those that had tackled the issue 'experientially', using 'real' cases with which trainees could identify. For example:

> When I went there I was expecting an in-depth approach, an educational view about AIDS, but it wasn't it was really about attitudes ... that was what I was looking for, it was helpful to learn things about attitude, you learn your own prejudices that you think you don't have, and then we had someone with full blown AIDS come in and talk to us all which was very moving ... (Nurse)

Indeed, the responses to training and education were overwhelmingly positive: virtually all respondents regarded it as having been helpful, both in terms of providing information and, perhaps more importantly, helping to allay fears or anxieties. The following were typical:

> It made you understand, it made you aware that there's not really any danger of actually getting it unless you have some sort of blood contact, so if you touch someone, or drink out of the same glass, there is no chance of getting it. I think it made me feel a lot better about HIV than I otherwise would have done. This leaflet backed up what the government said ... (Secretary, charity)

> Very useful because through my employment it's the only way I've known about it. Being employed in social services I've learnt a lot more than in general. Well I suppose because when we first knew about AIDS, it was all shock, horror, we're all going to catch it. But when you know more about it you find you're not so afraid. (Secretary, social services)

There are, however, two important cautions to be made about the provision of information and training. First, there was a clearly emerging scepticism on the part of many respondents towards generalized public health information campaigns; these were seen either as too abstract or tainted by apparent disagreement between 'experts'. In several cases, for instance, there was a high sensitivity to inconsistency in the 'official' message, as one respondent explained:

> the only qualm I'd have is that professional opinion seems to change from time to time, like we are seeing now, the forecast of heterosexual AIDS. The prediction of masses of people being infected has not started to happen. So obviously you take everything with a pinch of salt. Professional opinion might change. (Local authority officer)

Secondly, there is a more practical concern with the provision of training, namely, what could be described as the danger of 'P(olitical) C(orrectness) fatigue':

> I've no objections to making it specifically AIDS but I think that people have to see it as part of a wider context. Already with race awareness they are coming in and saying do you think I am racist, is that why I am going on the course. So they will either come in and say do you think I've got AIDS or do you think I've got a problem with people who have AIDS. (Manager, local authority)

Thus, although most respondents had gleaned an understanding of the 'big picture' of AIDS, there was a surprising uniformity in the lack of assurance with which respondents approached the issue at the level of practice. To the extent that many respondents realised the deficiencies in their understanding and expressed a desire for access to more and better training and education, a case can be made for the extension of such resources. However, the very ambivalence of many of the responses suggests that, even with such information, a constructive outcome, whilst clearly possible, is not inevitable.

Conclusion

It seems on a range of evidence that the predominant form in which members of an organization perceive and experience HIV/AIDS is as a dilemma. The exact nature of such dilemmas, however, is variable both in terms of the salience and impact of the choices involved. Thus, for most people with HIV, the choices relating to employment have a complex emotional loading and are likely to exercise a significant impact on both their physical and psychological well-being. For many of those not, as yet, affected by the epidemic, the employment issues associated with HIV/AIDS can appear to be of little *immediate* relevance but, on reflection, offer little prospect of easy resolution. Although formal policy is often seen as one means of pre-empting or resolving these dilemmas, it is unlikely that it can ever be wholly successful in this respect. The very logic of formal policy is to subordinate emotion to rationality, a logic which raises two significant issues. Firstly, there must be a question over the extent to which the relationship between rationality and emotion can be treated as a zero-sum game in which one can be used to drive out the other. As the previous chapter has shown, the mere existence of a policy does not guarantee that it will be adhered to in practice. Similarly, making available 'rational' prescriptions for attitudes and behaviour does not mean that emotional responses will be 'eliminated'. As our data has shown, many people may be less than convinced by the reassuring messages of 'experts', preferring to view the ramifications of HIV-infection with a strong sense of scepticism (see also Marquet *et al*, 1995). It is clearly unsatisfactory to dismiss such a lack of trust as mere irrationality borne out of ignorance that can be rectified by more 'facts'. Although lack of knowledge plays a considerable part in the uncertainty that undermines trust in expert discourses, other social factors will also be at work. Marquet *et al* (op cit), for instance, distinguish between 'distant mistrust' and 'vigilant mistrust'. The latter is defined as a mistrust borne out of a scepticism of the experts' 'real' understanding of the dynamics of HIV, characterized by the view that 'They say it isn't possible but I'm not so sure'. In Marquet *et al*'s research (based on a large survey of Belgians), vigilant mistrust was also associated with a relatively good factual understanding of HIV/AIDS, i.e., it was not simply a function of ignorance. In our own research this type of response was not uncommon among those who were relatively well informed, but it also took on another dimension more specific to the workplace and manifested in a mistrust of management's will to act 'fairly' in the treatment of people with HIV/AIDS if this potentially compromised any organizational interests. This form of mistrust was evidenced even in organizations which had constructive policies.

Distant mistrust, in contrast, is characterized as stemming from a more general scepticism based upon a relative lack of knowledge sustained by a sense of 'detachment' from 'experts and their world'. This view, which Marquet *et al* found to be more common among the 'culturally underprivileged', can be seen as being supported by a conservative and traditional sense of social identity and propriety that views outsiders (i.e., those 'not like us', which may include middle class, liberal experts and unashamed social 'deviants' such as homosexuals and drug-users) as objects of threat and repulsion. Again, there were some members of our study who seemed to adopt this stance, exhibiting both a distrust of expert opinion (including that contained in managerial policies) and of those perceived to be associated with HIV/AIDS.

The existence of these forms of mistrust, which in their intense subjective embeddedness in individual consciousness can be regarded as emotional, clearly pose difficulties for organizations wishing to develop constructive responses to HIV/AIDS. For, whereas a defensive response implicitly sustains both forms of mistrust, the fostering of a sustainable constructive practice demands that issues relating to HIV/AIDS are addressed not merely in formal terms, but also at a level that engages with a range of organizational issues and interests that go beyond the management of a medical condition and intersect with established power relations. One of the most crucial of these sets of power relations for responses to HIV/AIDS focuses around sex, sexuality and sexual orientation, and it is to a consideration of these issues that the next chapter is devoted.

Chapter 5

Sex, Work and HIV/AIDS

Introduction

The issue of AIDS cannot be separated from persisting inequalities of power and influence that pervade societies and organizations. Although involving inequalities of race, disability and class, the issue that has emerged most strongly in the HIV/AIDS debate is that of sex and sexuality, although significantly in most formal organizational responses this matter has been largely silent. Hearn and Parkin (1987, p. 81), however, talk of 'organization sexuality' by which they mean a 'sexual structuring' whereby organizations are continually divided by sex and sexualities, one characteristic of which is the dominance of male constructions of heterosexuality over other forms of sexuality. For them:

> The dominant concrete form that heterosexuality takes in this society is an hierarchical one. Thus a major, and perhaps central, feature of the sexual 'normality' of organizations is a powerful heterosexual bias: a form of 'compulsory heterosexuality' ... the domination and oppression of homosexuality, lesbianism and other sexualities perceived as 'other'. (Hearn and Parkin, 1987, p. 94)

In many organizations, however, this sexual configuration, whilst omnipresent, is not openly acknowledged; on the contrary, Burrell (1984) points to a pressure in formal policy and practice towards the de-sexualization of many modern forms of organization. AIDS, though, has impinged suddenly and unexpectedly upon the established sexual configuration of organization. Not only has it drawn attention to issues of sexual orientation and homosexual rights, but it has also made visible wider aspects of organization sexuality. On the one hand, it has drawn the sex industry and sex workers out of the shadows that have conveniently concealed them from public acknowledgment; and on the other, it reinforces the disadvantaged situation of many women in terms of their restricted access to jobs, wages and associated benefits.

Sex Work and the Sex Industry

Although the issues of HIV/AIDS and male homosexuality have been important axes of debate and struggle within conventional employing organizations such as businesses and public bodies, this should not lead to the neglect of those forms of employment that operate outside or on the margins of the conventional organizational arena. One such area where HIV/AIDS have become a particular issue is sex work, in particular prostitution.

Traditionally, sex work has been ignored by students of work and organization, reflecting a wider conspiracy of silence over its existence and the unwillingness of 'respectable' society to acknowledge its own demand for the service that sex workers provide (Plant, 1990). This silence has been compounded by the fact that, in the UK at least, prostitution takes place in the so-called black economy, is effectively if not technically criminal, and both emotionally and practically challenging as the site of empirical research (see, Plant, op cit; Patton, 1994, ch.3; Bury *et al*, 1992). Thus, research into sex work has remained located primarily in the sphere of social policy and, until recently, was usually defined solely as a social problem rather than being viewed as a form of employment or occupation. However, regardless of its legal status, prostitution is for significant numbers of women and men a source of work, either full or part-time, in which they may be engaged, albeit in some cases reluctantly, for considerable periods of their lives. These occupational characteristics are illustrated in Davies and Simpson's (1990) account of the different services offered by male prostitutes:

> The escort works for an agency, which takes a proportion of his earnings and offers a full range of sexual services in his own home or that of the client ... The masseur, by contrast, is self-employed and while he too provides a full service in his own or the client's home, he is also required to practice the trade of his

title ... Street-walking, as the name suggests, is a more casual occupation in the sense that it does not require the paraphernalia of telephones, advertisements and premises before clients are contacted. (1990, p. 114)

However, there are also aspects of sex work that expose its practitioners to greater risks of HIV infection than is the case with most other jobs (which is not to say that sex workers contribute to the spread of HIV to a greater extent than any other person, see below). According to Davies and Simpson (op cit), the role of prostitutes 'as a class' in HIV infection is somewhat analogous to that of health workers, but 'whereas the likelihood of, say, a nurse becoming infected in the normal course of duty is low, that of the prostitute is appreciably higher' (1990, p. 118). Prostitutes, in fact, often place themselves in situations where there is a potentially significant risk of transmission, whereas for the health worker, accidental transfusion with HIV positive blood is the only real risk of contracting the virus. For the prostitute, 'many if not all transactions carry at least the possibility of semen to blood contact' (ibid, p. 118).

Indeed, the assumption that 'prostitutes spread AIDS' has gained considerable currency in the popular media and in some professional circles, leading to sex workers having been identified early in the epidemic as a major potential vector for HIV transmission:

The most disturbing aspect of this is that the focus has been directed at sex workers with the underlying assumption that most, if not all, sex workers have AIDS, and if they have not already got 'IT', that they are not interested in preventing themselves from becoming infected. Attention and fear have centred around female sex workers infecting 'members of the general public', that is, 'normal' heterosexual males and thereby their 'normal' heterosexual partners. It would appear that clients bear no responsibility for their actions and are merely victims of the 'evil and predatory' sex workers. (Morgan Thomas, 1992, p. 72)

However, in terms of infection among prostitutes in Europe and the USA, the principal source seems to be injecting drug use or unprotected sex with partners who may also be injecting drug users. There is, in fact, considerable variation in the level of infection among prostitutes that seems to vary on a geographical basis associated with patterns of drug use in different urban cultures (Morgan Thomas, 1990; Kinnell, 1991; Plant, 1990). There is now considerable evidence to suggest that, given a real choice, most sex workers are prepared and anxious to use condoms and other prophylactics in the practice of commercial sex (Morgan Thomas, 1992; Scambler and Graham-Smith, 1992; Kinnell, op cit; Butcher, 1994). Although there is very little evidence of the spread of HIV from prostitute to client (Alexander, 1988), many clients do seem prepared to seek unprotected sex with prostitutes, thereby putting the prostitute and themselves at risk. Under the conditions in which sex work is conducted this demand from clients can severely limit the choices available to sex workers to protect themselves. As Morgan Thomas explains:

> Much has been made of the fact that some sex workers are willing to engage in unprotected sex for more money ... It is necessary to examine the degree of choice the sex worker has. Is it really greed on the part of the sex worker as depicted by many people, or are there other external factors at play? When a drug-addicted sex worker is offered more money — or 'double or nothing' — for unsafe sex, where is her choice if she needs her next 'fix'? When a woman has to pay the management for each client she receives, regardless of whether she receives any money, where is her choice? The choice is that of the client who is demanding unsafe sex. (Morgan Thomas, 1992, p. 79)

The ability to negotiate safe sex with clients is not a uniform process and some sex workers may find themselves in weaker bargaining positions than others. Morgan Thomas (above) points to some of the factors that restrict the choice of female prostitutes; Kinnell (op cit, p. 92) also points to the role that the 'setting' for sex work plays, her research in Birmingham having shown that women working in 'off-street' environments were more likely to have experienced sexual risk-taking with clients than street-workers. Hickson *et al*'s (1994, p. 206) study of male masseurs and escorts, however, suggests that these off-street workers appear to be relatively successful in maintaining a very high level of condom use with clients, especially casual ones. Although the experience of the prostitute (Davies and Simpson, 1990, p. 118) may play a part in these negotiations, it is also likely that culturally established differences in power between men and women also contribute. Female prostitutes are likely to find that the 'safer' environment (for the client) of off-street sex allows men to assert their traditional expectation of female submission to male 'desire' more easily than the uncertain and precarious locations of street sex where interruption and disturbance (by police and, increasingly, local vigilante groups) makes 'negotiation' (or insistence) difficult for the client. Ironically, because the expectation of deference between males is not so culturally fixed, the more obvious precariousness of the street-worker's condition may place him at a disadvantage with the client that is not always available within the more negotiable context of off-street sex (although Robinson and Davies' (1991) research would seem to question this, especially where younger streetworkers are desperate for accommodation).

In addition, the very nature of sex work may mean that prostitutes are less inclined to use condoms in their non-paying sexual relationships even though they will try to use them with their paying clients, a finding that appears to apply to both male and female prostitutes (Hickson *et al*, op cit; Kinnell, op cit). This is because the condom represents not only a means of protection against sexually transmitted diseases but also 'a physical barrier, a metaphor of exclusion for the woman at work, keeping the punter symbolically as far away as possible' (Butcher, op cit, p. 154). Ironically, possession of condoms by a woman suspected by police as being a prostitute may be used as evidence against her.

Although sex work may have many parallels with other forms of 'conventional' work, it also has significant differences stemming from its location as part of a black economy, the stigmatized perception of those who provide the services, their often limited power in shaping the conditions and terms of their employment, and the non-existence of any practical means by which abuse, maltreatment or exploitation can be exposed and remedied by legal means.

Thus, sex work draws attention to the limits of formal responses to HIV/AIDS regarded as best practice in other employment contexts. These latter depend to a significant extent upon the existence of bureaucratic employment procedures in which the basic rights and expectations of employees and employers are formally acknowledged and where some form of benign regulation is operable. Even where sex work comes close to conventional forms of contractual employment relationship, as with escorts, masseurs, club operators etc., the collusions of both employer and employee in an at best semi-legal activity is likely to render calls to formal, let alone legal, duties irrelevant. And in other areas of this industry sex workers may operate either as self-employed — but again with a positive incentive not to formalise any aspect of their working life (including their own health needs) for fear that this will facilitate prosecution — or in 'employment relationships' based on physical coercion or emotional manipulation rather than the instrumental rationality of the conventional contract.

However, it is not only in the 'black economy' of sex work that the unequal distribution of employment rights can influence the experience of HIV and AIDS. This is particularly the case with women's employment.

Women, HIV and Employment

The structural characteristics of women's employment are likely to mean that should they contract HIV their chances of constructive and supportive responses from an employer are potentially limited. The principal reason for this is the concentration of women either in low grade full-time jobs or in part-time employment. Indeed, in many instances women move from the former to the latter as they attempt to combine the role of sole or shared breadwinner with child-rearer and unpaid domestic worker (Dale, 1987; Hakim, 1994).

If, as Cockburn (1991) suggests, patriarchal capitalism 'defines women in domesticity', it is not surprising that their roles outside the household continue to be regarded by male employers and by some women as secondary or subsidiary to the principal role of mother/ housewife, a prioritising that is reflected in significantly worse terms and conditions of employment (Abercrombie and Warde, 1994; Dale, op cit). As Ginn and Arber (1993) argue in the case of occupational pensions:

> for most women career breaks, relatively low pay and long spells of part-time employment are common and likely to remain so in the absence of improved childcare and eldercare policies. Thus women with a domestic role will continue to form the bulk of early leavers and to earn lower occupational pensions than men. (Ginn and Arber, 1993, p. 67).

This argument extends more generally to the case of part-time women workers who, in the UK at present, often enjoy neither pro-rata wage rates nor full access to fringe benefits, such as pensions, sick leave, health insurance, holiday entitlement, etc. Even in the case of women with full-time employment, entitlement to such benefits may be significantly reduced by career breaks due to child rearing.

Given these generally disadvantageous entitlements and conditions of employment, it seems probable that women will often fare less well than men with HIV, even in companies adopting constructive responses, because of their relatively marginal position. For example, the typical constructive policy involves a commitment to maintain 'normal company rules regarding sick leave', but for women concentrated in lower grades or on part-time or temporary contracts this may be either limited or non-existent. They are more likely to be forced on to relatively low levels of state sickness benefit rather than enhanced occupational scheme payments, or if they do receive the latter, to receive lower amounts for shorter periods (because of lower levels or discontinuous contribution levels) than most men. It is also likely that managements concerned primarily with uninterrupted performance will resist providing adequate sickness leave to part-time or low level workers who are viewed as a dispensable resource. This is often exacerbated by the belief that women have not invested in 'serious' careers such that sickness does not need to be managed sympathetically (Hakim, 1992). Indeed, the structuring of part-time and temporary work is almost always shaped by the needs of the employer and not of the employee. While it may give the former considerable flexibility, it usually does not do so for the employee: although not necessarily conforming to 'normal' working hours, part-time work is generally extremely inflexible when it comes to employees wanting to adjust or change their working-time patterns. Under these conditions 'secondary' workers who are ill for more than a short period may well be pressured into abandoning work altogether, a strategy which managers can justify on the grounds that alternative part-time work is easily found and that, for women, it is an additional rather than a main income.

In these respects, then, many women who contract HIV and become ill are likely to find a lack of organizational support to allow them to continue working. Despite their wishes women in other than relatively secure occupational positions may be driven on to state benefit as the difficulties and stresses in maintaining a job in the face of lack of support, or even active discouragement, take a greater toll on health than remaining employed. The experiences of other disabled women in the labour market, for instance, give little reason for optimism. According to Lonsdale (1990):

> People with disabilities are at a serious disadvantage compared to the rest of the population in the labour market. They are less likely to have paid work. Thirty-three per cent of men with disabilities and 29 per cent of women with disabilities are in paid employment . . . while all people with disabilities are less likely to be employed, both disabled and non-disabled women are even less likely to be than their male counterparts . . . women being less likely to return to employment after the onset of disability. One study found 44 per cent of women returning to work, compared to 70 per cent of men. (Lonsdale, 1990, pp. 98–9)

In part, this reflects not only the inability or unwillingness of employers to structure work around the needs of ill or disabled people (see, chapter 3 above) but also an apparent expectation on the part of doctors and other 'experts' that for ill or disabled women, gaining employment is less of a priority — both for them and society in general — than it is for men (Lonsdale, op cit, p. 100). Thus, although there is little empirical research into the employment experiences of women with HIV, neither is there any encouraging evidence to suggest that it will follow a significantly different pattern from the experiences of women's employment in general and those of disabled women in particular. Indeed, experience of medical and governmental responses to women with HIV are less than encouraging, showing a pronounced pattern of marginalisation and lack of urgency (Patton, 1994, p. 12; Wilton, 1992, p. 50).

Compounding this structural disadvantage, however, is the cultural expectation that women will interrupt their employment to care for others, especially those to whom they are related. This expectation means that it is not only women who are themselves HIV positive who will have their employment opportunities affected but also those in a relationship with someone else who has the virus (which is not to say that an HIV positive woman will not also be expected to care for an infected relation). Although it must be recognised that this caring role has been taken by many men, especially members of the gay community through mechanisms such as buddying, there remains a stronger social expectation that such duties are more 'naturally' women's work. As Wilton points out:

It is women who take children to the dentist, the optician or the clinic for their check-ups and vaccinations, women who take time off work to care for sick children, women who look after their sick male partners, women who care for elderly or disabled relatives. Additionally women make up the greater part of the volunteer workforce . . . Even at the Terrence Higgins Trust, Britain's most important AIDS service organization, over half the volunteers are women, despite the facts that the majority of the HIV positive clients served by the Trust are men and that the Trust has its roots in the gay male community. (Wilton, 1992, p. 50)

This is also recognized by Altman (1994, p. 19) who speaks of the 'double impact' of HIV on women: that is, as being at greater risk of infection and those upon whom the burden of care falls most heavily. For many women in work this is likely to mean that they will feel obliged (and be expected) to disrupt their careers, to renegotiate their hours, or to give up working altogether to care for a partner, child, or parent who has become ill through HIV. And, as a result, they may limit their access to pension rights, sick leave for themselves should they fall ill, and since they will most likely be forced into part-time or temporary work, benefits such as compassionate leave that remain largely the prerogative of full-timers and higher grades. HIV/AIDS, of course, is not unique in causing this effect, but it is another issue that needs highlighting in the face of the still widely held assumption that women are not greatly affected by the epidemic. In this case, as well, the effects will be felt not only in the sacrifices made at the time of caring, but also later in life through limited pension and benefit support.

HIV/AIDS, Homosexuality and Workplace Attitudes

However, despite the prospect of increasing infection and the limited prospects facing women affected by HIV, it remains a fact that in the UK four out of five cases of AIDS are among gay men, and over 13,000 are HIV positive — compared to 3,000 women in 1994. As Dockrell (1994, p. 28) has pointed out: 'Heterosexual transmission is the fastest growing route of transmission but ... for every new heterosexual infection there are two new gay infections'. Reflecting this, the bulk of recorded cases of discrimination against people with HIV have been associated, directly or indirectly, with attitudes towards homosexuality (see, chapter 6 below for a fuller discussion of the legal implications).

In 1987, for example, the airline Dan Air was censured by the Equal Opportunities Commission for its policy of not recruiting male cabin staff, a policy that it tried to justify on the grounds that over 30 per cent of male applicants for such posts were gay and that, as HIV affected (gay) men to a greater extent than women, their employment might pose a health risk to passengers.

The case of Buck vs Letchworth Palace Ltd. (1987) involved a gay man who was dismissed after colleagues discovered from a local newspaper that he had been convicted of gross indecency. They then refused to work with him on the grounds that having to share toilet and canteen facilities put them at risk of contracting HIV. Management conceded to their demands and dismissed the man, additionally justifying their action on the grounds of needing to protect children who might visit the cinema where the man had been employed — apparently confirming the stereotype of gay men as incorrigible child-molesters.

A London Law centre dismissed two solicitors for having maliciously harassed a new solicitor who had previously worked for the gay Switchboard on the grounds that he would introduce AIDS into the organization (Philpott vs N Lambeth Law Centre, 1986). Research by Ross (1993) in the USA provides further examples of this so-called 'co-categorisation' effect whereby revelation of being HIV positive also exposes a gay identity which, in turn, can lead to discrimination and/or insensitive and hurtful comments and jokes relating both to homosexuality and HIV (p. 209), resulting in involuntary or pressured job changes.

Thus, the early characterization of HIV/AIDS as the 'gay plague' has meant that it carries with it a constant reference of homosexuality (Watney, 1989; Weeks, 1991:ch. 6) such that it threatens to disrupt the established principles of organization sexuality. The remainder of this chapter sets out to examine this potential for disruption in more detail, in particular to explore the ways in which understandings of HIV/AIDS are linked by organization members to notions of sexuality. The data presented is taken from our own research (see chapter 4 above for details) with the intention of providing insights into these issues through the use of qualitative data. It is hoped that this data, while not statistically representative, will point to the complexities and contradictions that underlie the formal approaches discussed in earlier chapters.

For the purposes of exposition we have organized our data via a typology of attitudes to AIDS developed by Herek and Glunt (1991).

This US research labels the axes of the typology Pragmatism/Moralism and Coercion/Compassion and defines their quadrants as follows.

First, the Compassionate Secularism pattern characterizes the general stance of the American public health community and of the lesbian and gay male community: endorsement of such non-moralistic pragmatic policies as distribution of condoms and sterile needles, as well as opposition to coercive measures such as quarantine. . . . Second, a pattern of Compassionate Moralism . . . is reflected in the official pronouncements of the Conference of Catholic Bishops: compassion is urged for people with AIDS, but education about condoms is rejected on moral grounds. . . . Third, Punitive Moralism, endorsement of coercive measures and rejection of non-moralistic pragmatic policies, is perhaps best exemplified in the US by spokespersons of conservative political and religious beliefs. . . . Indiscriminate Action . . . may reflect an acquiescent response set [and] considerable ambivalence concerning AIDS: views of people with AIDS as both dangerous and deserving of compassion . . . containment as well as pragmatic education and prevention. (cited in Pollack *et al*, 1992, p. 28)

The criteria we use to allocate cases to categories have been developed inductively from our data to reflect the specific focus on sexual identity in the workplace while retaining the sense of Herek and Glunt's original categories. The distribution of respondents between these categories is given in fig. 1. These criteria are outlined at the beginning of each sub-section.

Figure 1. Herek and Glunt's Typology of attitudes to AIDS

Compassionate

COMPASSIONATE MORALISM (10)	COMPASSIONATE SECULARISM (10)
Moralistic ———————————	————————— Pragmatic
PUNITIVE MORALISM (6)	INDISCRIMINATE ACTION (8)

Coercive

N = 34 (only those respondents who explicitly mentioned sexuality related issues are included in this analysis, no respondent appears in more than one category)

Compassionate Secularism

In ideal-typical terms Compassionate Secularism is represented by beliefs which:

1 embody a commitment not to discriminate unfairly against people affected by HIV/AIDS;

2 recognise the importance of heterosexism as an additional basis for discrimination that may be attached to AIDS;

3 demonstrate a commitment to gaining greater acceptance — ideally parity — of non-heterosexual identities and the lengthening of the equal opportunities agenda.

A principal concern of those falling into this category was an acute awareness of the potential for prejudice resulting from misconceived links between AIDS and homosexuality. Thus, when speaking of the issues to which AIDS could give rise in the workplace, most drew attention to the pervasiveness of homophobia. For example:

> I remember at a board meeting in my previous company a manager was almost passed over because of being gay, not because of his ability but because the way the guy wanted to live his life. But because somebody said he was gay they thought, 'Hang on fellows, what are we talking about?' The argument that ensued was quite interesting because then they started looking at other guys' behaviours, far more damning because the gay guy was very discreet, kept his private life very private and performed his job and was well respected and a good manager. Another colleague who was 'one of the boys', was in fact often an acute embarrassment because of his drinking and womanising. But he was 'okay' and this was from board level guys. So you've got a lot of prejudice and stereotyping. (Hotel Personnel Manager)

> We did do an exercise once about prejudice and how we could perceive people to be. You get the young looking hairdresser and we did a group and they said he must be gay because he is a hairdresser and he is young and that's how we have perceived that person to be and yet we can be so wrong so many times and I think it's a shame. (Personnel Manager retail/distribution)

I think it's sexuality that is the problem for people and I don't think people know it. Its mixed into a lot of fear and misunderstanding about HIV and I think in terms of employing somebody with HIV, I still think most people are at the point where HIV comes along with a panic and you don't know how to control it. So I think certainly it's an issue around sexual orientation, I think people have their personal prejudices around that and how they manage that. (Social Worker)

Given this awareness of heterosexual bias as a factor influencing reactions to AIDS, respondents frequently pointed to the need for education about associated sexual attitudes and values, thus:

The THT 'Positive Management' pack was very well done. I particularly liked the non-detrimental scenario that they were putting out, very real dealing with everyday people. Characters that they were using, ordinary looking people, everyday kinds of people saying things clearly, it kind of brought it home. I showed it to other people, it's almost like you were confronted with it and suddenly it raised an awful lot of questions like, 'I would never have believed that guy was gay?'; 'What's he supposed to have? Three heads?', this kind of thing. It's getting rid of the stereotypes. (Hotel Personnel Manager)

Our experience of talking about issues of HIV and AIDS means you are talking about love and sex and all of those things which people don't tend to talk about at work. Quite a lot of barriers were broken down when we started having those conversations and I think it created a good feeling and brought us closer to each other as a result, but that was nearly a year ago. Maybe we need to do something to get that closeness back. (Distribution Manager)

The course was held in London, that was actually presented by a chap who was gay and his partner who in fact was HIV positive, which they did not divulge until near the end, that really went in to more how people feel. That was very useful ... They were very good and effective. (Personnel Manager, Charity)

However, despite a certain consistency, this category was by no means completely homogeneous, tending to divide between those who favoured a 'low key' and informal resolution of the AIDS-sexuality dilemma, and those who advocated open confrontation and formalization. The former response was summed up by the hotel personnel manager who began by pointing to the complexities surrounding homosexual identities in heterosexually structured organizations:

> I think that the most important thing is that people have got to feel okay. There are members of the gay community who are very comfortable with their sexuality and don't give a damn. There is another group which are comfortable but are not so open and there are some who are very scared and they are often fearful of what would happen if it became common knowledge that they were gay and it acts like an extra burden to carry. They assume people automatically think if they are gay then they assume they are HIV positive. (Hotel Personnel Manager)

For this respondent the important aspect of dealing with AIDS and sexuality in the workplace was to establish a culture of trust in which all organization members would be treated as individuals and assessed on their job performance rather than on the basis of their social 'status'. This led to a scepticism towards the effectiveness of rule-making and formal policy:

> I am concerned about making any policy illness-related as in the majority of cases in our company primarily one group of people, which is the gay people, will be affected. Any legislation which focuses on one particular social group I have a problem with. It refocuses the mind on the wrong points. (Hotel Personnel Manager)

Here, sexuality was considered a matter of private identity that should properly be separate from work *role* (although not necessarily completely subsumed by a workplace *identity*). Thus, where an identity-role conflict occurred this could be dealt with on a case-by-case basis within a framework of tolerance. As this respondent explained:

> One experience I have had that was memorable, it surprised everybody ... The initial reaction was shock, horror and the disbelief that Nigel was gay. Then some embarrassment, then

some guilt, like 'Why he didn't tell us?' then it goes back to shock again, because then you realise that he has got HIV and potentially that he could be dead in a certain length of time. Then there is a tremendous feeling of 'What can we do?' When the guy did die the reaction from the staff was considerable. (Hotel Personnel Manager)

In this case, it seems, compassion is personal and individual, and secularism implies expurgation of sexuality from *formal* organization discourse. This stance parallels the notion of 'hidden conflict' (Kolb and Putnam, 1992) whereby some issues are dealt with informally and privately and resolved by 'avoidance, accommodation, tolerance or behind-the-scenes coalition building' rather than confrontation (1992, p. 19). However, while such a strategy can be justified on the grounds that, given existing disparities in sex-power, it is better to 'bend with the wind' than to 'snap in the breeze', it could also be objected to because it appears to acquiesce in the dominance of heterosexism (see, Cockburn, 1991).

Indeed, for another respondent, this strategy of informal accommodation was less attractive than a frontal challenge to established heterosexism. AIDS, in fact, was seen as a weapon in the attempt to gain organizational acceptance of homosexual identity:

The equal opps policy is on the grounds of race, gender, physical ability, religion, leaves out sexual orientation and HIV status which is a terrible error, terrible omission, there's massive resistance to AIDS ... I think its a good way to get sexual orientation considered actually. I know a lot of places wouldn't normally consider that in their equal opps scheme but have as a result of having to consider HIV status ... the drawbacks are that it emphasizes feelings like the gay plague type of thing, but that's not a drawback in the long term. As long as sexual orientation gets in there, I'm not really bothered about how as long as it does. As long as its in there they can't damn you for it. (Social Worker)

This latter stance placed a greater emphasis on formal recognition of homosexualities, including sanctions against those who proved maliciously recalcitrant, and emphasised a commitment that this issue should be faced openly and collectively, as a social rather than a purely personal matter.

Indiscriminate Action

Indiscriminate Action, like Compassionate Secularism, retains a focus that is pragmatic rather than moralistic but combines this with an acceptance of coercive measures against people with HIV/AIDS. Thus, it involves:

1 an ambivalence towards AIDS with particular views informed by specific circumstances and situations;
2 a 'common sense' view that homosexuality is a credible associate of HIV infection and, as such, those claiming (or suspected of having) such an identity can legitimately be treated with suspicion;
3 a preparedness to accept discriminatory measures if there is felt to be any chance of risk to the 'healthy' population; where no such risk is apparent a strategy of 'live and let live/die' may be adopted.

The concept of Indiscriminate Action reflects an ostensibly amoral stance guided by concerns of prudent self-protection in the face of an uncertain hazard (Smithurst, 1990). In one case, for instance, the issue of sexual transmission was presented as a *universal* threat rather than a matter of moral distaste, which justified HIV testing on a grand scale and workplace surveillance of sexual behaviour:

I think something ought to be done worldwide as regards the testing of AIDS, its a very serious thing. I think everyone should be tested, it's a frightening thing, ... [If I thought someone was HIV positive] I would be wary of the fact, and keep an eye on his/her behaviour, it's like if he or she started sleeping around, you know. (Nightclub Manager)

In other cases, though, the links between AIDS, risk and sexuality were configured in terms which implicated homosexuality as an object of concern if not explicit moral condemnation. For example:

I don't see anything against homosexuals or anything like that, but I think we ought to know, we need to be more careful about it. But they are not the only ones who carry AIDS, I mean there is a hell of a lot of other groups who carry AIDS. (Metal Worker A)

This association of AIDS and homosexuality, however, did have a bearing on the sorts of 'action' which were considered appropriate for workplace settings. A benign form, for instance, involved a management decision deliberately to exclude AIDS from equal opportunities policy agendas in order to forestall raising questions of sexual orientation, this suppression of homosexual identity being justified pragmatically because of its perceived threat to other 'mainstream' policies. Thus:

> We haven't really addressed the area of equal opps relating to sexuality and AIDS. It's not something we want to raise, not because we don't want to, but we don't want to be diverted from a number of other things which we are still having to argue issues about. I mean we shouldn't have to argue women's issues in 1993. If we got diverted and we know there's going to be a lot of objections, it's not going to help the equal opps policy, so we haven't addressed sexual health issues in the equal opps policy so far. (Public Sector manager)

Similar, but less clearly articulated, negative associations between homosexual identity and HIV-infection were also made by employees in health-care organizations. Here, too, the issue was one of individual tolerance outweighed by perceived disruption to organizational operations:

> If members of the public found out that somebody here was HIV positive or that we were seeing AIDS patients, our practice would lose patients, I know it would. There is still a stigma attached to it. It's still the gay plague. (Dental Assistant)

> If they are a student, part of their training is how to give injections, and they go to do a bit of practice and there is a mishap, you have an injury, and there is your problem. I think the answer is that, I suppose there is no reason why they could not do the academic part of the course, but I don't know about the practical . . .
> We have a [gay] lad at the moment and he is lovely and the way he talks to families, he *actually* gets on quite well now. I mean *as people* they have been very nice. (Nurse)

Note in the last quotation the unstated identification of the gay man as 'other than a normal person'. The question of whether this 'otherness' includes propensity to be HIV positive thus remains open and, as such, creates at least the potential for action to be discriminatory.

Indeed, other responses involved the open approval of surveillance and 'investigation' applied to employees known to be or suspected of being gay, although as one noted, it was 'nothing personal'. For example:

> I mean you'd want to go into their personal lives to find out if he is a homo or if this particular person does sleep around without the proper precautions. (Metal Worker B)

> Maybe on the gay side, asking them maybe to have a urine test to make sure they haven't contracted during the time. (Hotel manager)

Responses in this category were not without their own tensions which, in the absence of a strong moral dimension, mostly hinged around issues of practicality. In particular, there was a 'resigned tolerance' whereby action against those perceived as likely 'carriers' of HIV was rejected on grounds of feasibility rather than principle. For instance:

> I don't think you would ever get a straight answer, certainly if you asked someone if they were a drug user. So I don't think you would ever get a straight answer if you ask somebody what their sexual persuasions are. (Hotel Manager)

> I don't know, how do you go about asking that sort of thing anyway? I don't think it is ever going to be one of those things you're going to be able to solve. (Metal Worker B)

There is clearly a problem in regarding the boundaries of this group too rigidly. It was apparent that in some cases, and despite claims of amorality, there was a strong sense of disapproval towards homosexuality, evidenced by one respondent thus:

> I personally haven't, this is my personal opinion, I haven't got any time for homosexuals, they leave me alone, I'll leave them alone. And er, no they just should be treated like the rest of us. No favouritism and no discrimination . . . I mean I've seen incidents and cases read about them, there was a column in the Sunday paper a couple of weeks ago where this journalist was stuck on a train full of homosexuals and they were being discriminative

against straight people and abusive. Nothing happened to them so why should anything happen to straight people if they are discriminative against them? (Metal Worker A)

It is quite possible, therefore, that this category may capture what respondents perceive to be 'respectable' answers, thereby masking views more appropriately classified as either Compassionate Moralism or Punitive Moralism.

Compassionate Moralism

Moving to the 'moral' side of the typology, Compassionate Moralism can be defined by:

1 a commitment not to discriminate unfairly against people affected by HIV/AIDS;

2 a belief that AIDS is largely the result of 'unnatural' or irresponsible behaviour, and that those affected are, thus, not wholly without blame for their condition;

3 the view that while those with AIDS/HIV should not be the subject of repressive control, neither should the behaviour responsible for their predicament be encouraged or openly condoned; in short, they should be viewed as deserving of pity and sympathy but not unconditional support.

A common theme among respondents in this category was a concern to establish a sense of difference between themselves and, as one quaintly put it, those of 'a homosexual persuasion'. For instance:

Now most people who are in a normal, god fearing working life, like you and I, I assume, we don't really come into heavy contact with people like that, do we? Homosexuals are very clandestine because of the nature of their relationships ... they don't live a normal life, as we know. (Metal Worker C)

Indeed, it was the ability to maintain this difference that provided the discursive space for expressions of tolerance and sympathy. Consider the following:

I used to like Queen [the rock group] and I thought 'Oh God! No, not him', because I think he [Freddy Mercury] was a real ..., you know, and then it put me off of his music. So it could put me off a person, that's what I am saying, I really used to like him, and then I thought, 'Oh goodness no, what a waste of a life', or whatever, but then again, how do you know how he caught it? (Print worker)

It is general knowledge that homosexuals obviously transmit it [HIV] through their varied, colourful sex life ... Not that I'm homosexual! ... But most of it is people who are a bit frightened of them because they don't really understand them. Now, what they are doing is not what was written in the good book, so therefore it must be wrong ... as long as they don't interfere with your life or in any way try to persuade you to their way of thinking then they should have the same rights as us, shouldn't they. (Metal Worker C)

I mean it was one of those things that I'd sort of put two and two together anyway just from observing him. I just had this gut feeling. You just sort of pick up vibes don't you, and I had thought he was perhaps homosexual anyway, er, he was always very pleasant, I just had that feeling. (Clerical Worker, Factory)

The last quotation picks up another theme in the maintenance of difference, namely its achievement — somewhat paradoxically — through exaggerated expressions of surprise about how 'normal' individual homosexuals were 'really' (often along the lines of 'some of my best friends are gay'). As others illustrate:

In Devon where I worked we had a gay bar man, he wasn't overtly gay he was in the closet and you know I got on fine with him, there were no problems. (Barman A, nightclub)

I went on a tour of Europe and one of the guys was gay, he didn't tell any of us, because he thought especially the guys, might think differently of him; and all the girls knew, I don't know his manner, just his way, I mean it didn't bother us. (Barman B, nightclub)

We have a gay at the moment in the coffee house and he's been there a long time about 18 years with the company. (Hotel Receptionist)

The quotations cited above can be seen as representing attempts by respondents to manage what were perceived to be the 'spoilt identities' of others (Goffman, 1963). However, although it has often been pointed out that defining others as deviant or abnormal can serve to reconfirm dominant standards of normality, the respondents here were not working with such a simple binary divide; rather, the normal/abnormal distinction appeared as a duality, a tension, between a 'virtual' and an 'actual' identity (ibid). It involved the assumption that a homosexual identity was essentially 'discredited' — doubly so given its association with AIDS — but that opportunities could be provided for such individuals to prove by their actions that *they* were not wholly so. In effect this meant the creation of the social space to allow a status transformation from discredited to discredit*able*, that is, the *potential* to be discredited, thereby enabling a tacit agreement to ignore — but not repudiate — the stigmatized identity, provided other expressions of 'normality' were maintained. Such a 'transformation' is facilitated by the implicit and explicit 'rules' that maintain organization sexualities (Mills and Murgatroyd, 1991). Thus, the acid-test for 'discreditability' is the extent to which these often unspoken rules are obeyed. This was highlighted in the accounts of respondents who recalled situations when the bounds of such propriety had been overstepped:

The only one we had here, we had a transvestite here, he was a nice looking chap but he liked to dress in the female dress, the only trouble was that he was using the women's toilet so we had to sack him. (Metal Worker C)

... if someone came in there, if somebody came in and talking like a madam and with a really high voice then they might pull jokes about him, that type of thing I mean. (Print Worker)

It seemed, then, that the precondition for the 'toleration of difference' was an individual deference towards heterosexual 'normality' on the part of the 'other' and a suppression of deliberate expressions of homosexuality.

Punitive Moralism

The final category, Punitive Moralism, rests upon the following:

1 AIDS is a disease resulting from fundamentally corrupt and perverse sexual behaviours;
2 those who have the virus, and are thus implicated in such behaviour, are both a medical and a moral threat to others and should, therefore, be excluded from normal social relations, including employment;
3 steps to identify and discriminate against such people both at the pre- and post-employment stage are defensible and desirable.

The general tenor of responses in this category reflected a more rigid view of the discredited homosexual identity as incapable of even partial 'redemption'. This is captured by the following quotations:

if I knew there was a homosexual here, then I would possibly, certainly protest slightly . . . I would turn around and I definitely wouldn't work with the person. It might sound nasty. I don't know whether I could accept it. It's like I suppose taking your child into a house where you know someone has HIV . . . with your own kid it's the last thing you'd want. (Chef, Public Sector)

They wouldn't work here. They would be fired straight away . . . there would just be an atmosphere in there all the time . . . I would keep away. (Nightclub Manager)

However, in addition to an antipathy towards homosexuality these respondents also tended to exhibit low levels of understanding of HIV and, to a greater extent than other respondents, felt themselves personally to be at risk from the virus (see, the quotations from some of these respondents relating to risk cited in chapter 4 above). In addition to framing these issues in terms of risk there was a tendency to locate them in relation to guilt and innocence. Thus, distinctions were made between those who were infected with HIV 'accidentally' and those who had contracted the virus as a result of 'unacceptable' and 'irresponsible' activity. Thus:

I've got a lot of sympathy for those who are heterosexual, but I haven't got much sympathy for homosexuals because they know what they are getting involved with ... I wouldn't want them touching me, well it's silly to say that, I would feel sorry for them depending totally on the circumstances ... If he was known to be very promiscuous, I wouldn't feel too sorry for him as he brought it on himself. (Nightclub waitress)

... you've got more chance of getting HIV if you are homosexual than heterosexual. I wouldn't like to be expert on homosexuality or like that ... But I think gays are a high risk and they should at least check it out ... I'm a clean person so I know I'm okay. (Nightclub Bouncer)

In our research such open expressions were a rarity but, as will be discussed below, such fears may be present in many respondents at a deeper level and be quite capable of being brought to the surface by particular incidents. However, neither are they dissimilar to accounts drawn from other organizations. For example, the response of a personnel manager to a course on AIDS-awareness run by a national AIDS charity illustrates this point:

I felt as if I had been hijacked by the AIDS lobby. Everyone in the group was all in favour of equality of sexual practices, and I felt I was in a minority of one seeing homosexuality as an unfortunate aberration and not approving of overt homosexuality ... (Johnstone, 1992, p. 45)

An even more extreme case is reported by Cockburn (1991):

I asked men [in High Street Retail (one of 4 case study firms)] ... if they thought it would be appropriate to add protection of the employment rights of homosexuals to their equality policy. Few had any inhibitions about voicing a resounding 'no'. 'It's wrong to foster these bent attitudes', 'they are spreading disease — it's not good for the nation or for the company' were views widely echoed. Others said, 'I'm not into these bloody weirdos, I just don't want to know', 'it's disgusting, turns my stomach', 'if you want to be "out", it's out *you* go as far as I'm concerned'. (Cockburn, 1991, p. 192, emphasis in original).

Indeed, as the accounts of workplace prejudice against homosexuals detailed in previous chapters have shown, the effects of discriminatory behaviour by a very small number of people — even a single individual — can be severe, especially if other organization members either 'turn a blind eye' or are prepared to collude passively in its exercise.

Conclusions

Through those activities which constitute the sex industry HIV poses, in effect, an occupational hazard that is now always potentially present in the practice of sex work. In most other forms of employment, however, where direct sexual contact is not part of the employment relationship — officially if not always unofficially — HIV/AIDS is still likely to be perceived through the twin lenses of gender and sexuality. Through the former there is likely to be a marginalization of its potential effects, reflecting, on the one hand, a general tendency for women's employment to be treated as secondary and, as such, attracting limited benefit entitlements and, on the other, the still pervasive view that HIV is not a 'real problem' for women. Such a view, of course, ignores both women's vulnerability to infection with HIV and the social expectation that women will 'normally' adopt the role of carer for partners or dependants who may fall ill with AIDS-related diseases (Wilton op cit). The definitions of organization sexuality also frame the understanding of HIV/AIDS and as our data suggest, these are largely constructed in terms of the normality of heterosexuality.

As the use of the typology demonstrated, however, within this general pattern the extent to which other sexualities were regarded as deviant or stigmatized was variable, a variability which, in turn, coloured potential responses to HIV/AIDS. Given this range of understandings it is possible to see how defensive responses can both be generated and sustained, offering supposedly simple solutions to these inherently difficult questions. Alternatively, however, there are also opportunities for constructive responses to be developed, particularly in a long agenda form which can address the associated issues around gender and sexual inequality. As was indicated in chapter three, however, the development of an effective constructive response within the context of employing organizations is neither automatic nor easy. Indeed, because such a strategy inevitably involves a challenge to existing distributions of power and resources within organizations, some level of resistance or challenge is inevitable — on economic if not 'moral' grounds. Such challenges have, of course, already been mounted in areas of sex and race equality (although these are still far from being won) where the adoption of legislation has been a principal means of providing both protection and remedy for disadvantaged groups. It is, therefore, necessary to examine to what extent this form of regulation currently influences the employment opportunities of people with HIV/AIDS and what prospects it might hold for the future.

Chapter 6

HIV/AIDS and British Employment Law

Introduction

The material presented in the foregoing chapters, while pointing to the complex nature of organizational responses to HIV/AIDS also confirms the real prospect of encountering workplace discrimination and prejudice — from employers and/or co-workers — as a result of HIV status (Harris and Haigh, 1990; Wilson, 1993; Wilson, 1994; Green, 1995). While the detriment suffered may be minimised by constructive employer action, for example, in the form of HIV/AIDS policies and education, this remains a choice for organizations since there is no specific British legislation designed to provide protection for these employees in the workplace. That legislation which does exist is primarily concerned with public health matters, three specific HIV/AIDS related measures being currently in force: the Public Health (Infectious Diseases) Regulations 1985 which make certain sections of the Public Health (Control of Disease Act) 1984 applicable to AIDS; the AIDS Control Act 1987; and the Health and Medicines Act 1988. The AIDS Control Act provides for the collection of statistics relating to HIV and AIDS while the 1988 Act has one Section aimed at preventing the sale of home HIV testing kits and the growth of fee testing establishments. It is, however, the first act that is perhaps the most interesting in that its provisions reflect the wide scale ignorance of HIV transmission at the beginning of the epidemic, and the level of panic which the disease induced. It allows local authorities to order the medical examination of a person with AIDS or who is HIV positive if it is 'in the interest of the individual, the family or the public generally' and provides for magistrates to issue a warrant to a police officer to enter premises in connection with the undertaking of such a medical examination. On the order of a magistrate, people with AIDS, but not those who are HIV positive, can be removed to, and detained in, a hospital if circumstances indicate that the patient will not take proper precautions to prevent the spread of infection. Other sections of these regulations concern the body of someone who has died as a result of AIDS: it not being allowed to keep the corpse in the home before burial or to allow viewing of the body in an open coffin. It can be noted in passing that it was this type of highly regulatory response, framed in medico-legal terminology, that provided the backdrop for the development of many defensive workplace responses (see, chapter 2 above) — especially in the field of health care — and was often reflected in the privileging of the right of management unilaterally to dictate and control the activities of organization members affected by HIV/AIDS.

The potential for discrimination in the workplace that HIV/AIDS engenders in the absence of specific legal provisions was, however, increasingly recognized during the 1980s, and towards the end of this period there were two attempts to introduce specific legislation on HIV/AIDS and employment. The first, in 1987, sought to make dismissal on the grounds of HIV infection or having AIDS (or suspicion of this) an inadmissible reason for dismissal, and was drafted from recommendations made to David Alton MP by the Terrence Higgins Trust. Modest in its aims, it specifically allowed an employer to dismiss if the employee was incapable of fulfilling the terms of the contract of employment, that is, the existing law (outlined below) concerning dismissal on the grounds of ill-health would still apply. The Bill was withdrawn when the Departments of Health and Employment could provide no evidence of discrimination against those with AIDS to the Bill's sponsor. The second, proposed by Gavin Strong MP as an amendment to the 1989 Employment Bill sought to make it unlawful to discriminate in the selection of employees, the provision of terms and conditions of employment and the dismissal of staff on the grounds that the person had contracted, or was believed to be at risk of contracting, HIV. Again, dismissal was not to be unfair if the employee was unable to perform the duties under the contract of employment. In the debate by the Bill's Standing Committee, the clause was defeated by the Conservative members of the Committee.

More recently, a further attempt to outlaw discrimination against those with HIV/AIDS was via the much publicized private member's Civil Rights (Disabled Persons) Bill, 1994. This had a 'three pronged' definition of disability, and in its application to employment matters appeared closely to mirror the provisions of the US Americans With Disabilities Act (see, chapter 7 below) to the extent that some of the latter's clauses were reproduced verbatim. Had it passed into legislation it would appear that as far as HIV/AIDS is concerned the Bill would have been expected to achieve the same objectives as the American Act, but it was 'talked out' in the House of Commons because the Government was persuaded that the costs of implementation were unaffordable. However, in response to the pressure for legislation generated by the lobby accompanying the Bill, the Government has drafted its own measure, the Disability Discrimination Bill 1995. This has a much narrower definition of disability than that contained in the previous private member's Bill and although it appears to offer limited protection to those who have developed AIDS, the position of those with asymptomatic HIV is unclear at this stage. In addition, the Bill does not apply to those employing fewer than 20 employees thus removing from its coverage some 95 per cent of UK firms.

Unlike the three earlier attempts at legislation, the Disability Discrimination Bill does not include any provision to make unlawful discrimination based on the *belief* (correct or not) of a person's HIV status. As earlier chapters have suggested, such beliefs may often arise out of simplistic and misinformed assumptions regarding a causal connection between homosexuality and HIV infection: addressing this issue exposes a weakness in existing legislation to which this chapter will return. However, until specific legislation is introduced what assistance the law can provide depends upon the application of existing acts of parliament and case law to the specific circumstances of an individual employee's complaint. Whether potential and existing employees with HIV/AIDS are able to use legal provisions to prevent or overcome unfair treatment from an employer, and the extent to which these provisions may shape organization responses, requires an understanding of how employment law may relate to the particular issues of HIV infection. The remainder of this chapter examines the applicability of existing employment law to HIV/AIDS and assesses its impact upon employment practice.

In Britain, the legal relationship between an employee and employer is based upon the concept of a contract of employment which contains the respective rights and duties of both parties. The contract remains a concept, however, since for most employees their contract is not contained in one single, written document. Rather, it is made up of a complex mixture of spoken and written terms and conditions of employment. In addition to any particular terms agreed by the employee and employer, judicial decisions have constructed a number of implied duties — 'common law terms' — owed by the parties to each other. While the principles on which these are based were developed in the last century, typically seen in the description of the parties as 'master' and 'servant' (Hepple, 1979), they remain powerful determinants of the behaviour of which the courts will approve.

Over the last three decades, the field of employment law has witnessed an expansion of statutory legislation designed to give specific protection to employees which extends and adds to that implicitly contained in the common law. This legislation covers areas as unfair dismissal, sex and race discrimination, maternity provisions and compensation for job loss in circumstances of redundancy. Significantly, much of the employment legislation introduced in the last fifteen years has been passed in order to meet Britain's obligations as a member of the European Community/Union. Specific measures originating in European law which may have a bearing on the employment position of those who are seropositive are discussed in chapter 7 below.

The Lack of Case Law

One difficulty in examining the application of employment law to cases involving HIV/AIDS is the relative absence of cases that have reached the courts. Given that various reports have documented a number of cases where employees have suffered some form of workplace detriment (Harris and Haigh, 1990; Wilson, 1992, 1994), it appears strange that this position has arisen. Indeed, Wilson (1992) reports that the experience of HIV advice agencies is that employment problems are the second most common type of enquiry from their clients. A number of possibilities may exist by way of explanation. First, the limited value of the law on discrimination and, to a lesser extent, unfair dismissal where there is a need to ensure the facts of the case fit legal definitions which were not designed to deal with HIV/AIDS specifically. Second, for cases of unfair dismissal an employee requires at least two years continuous service with an employer before being qualified to bring a claim. Thus, employees working in sectors where labour turnover is high are less likely to be able to meet the service criterion. Third, the psychological impact of the attendant publicity which tribunal cases may attract, particularly in such 'newsworthy' matters as AIDS, and which may mean that, even if successful in the case, dismissed employees may have difficulty finding other employment. Finally, those who have developed AIDS may find the stress attached to mounting a claim sufficiently severe to make the exercise not worthwhile.

In her study of the advice given to those with HIV/AIDS by voluntary agencies, Wilson (1993) argues that the last two factors, publicity and stress, can be significant in explaining the dearth of cases going to court. These, she suggests, lead many non-legally trained advisors to regard the law as a less than useful mechanism for resolving problems arising from HIV infection. She quotes the views of two advisors in her study, the first commenting on the impact of publicity and the other highlighting the effects of stress:

> ... the bottom line is unless you are prepared for the whole world to find out you've got AIDS there is nothing you can do, your only legal remedy in many cases is to take your employer to industrial tribunal. Industrial tribunals are not held in secret, and if you go to tribunal and allege you were sacked because of AIDS you run the risk of that appearing on the front page of your local newspaper and most people are just not prepared to run that risk and I can't say I blame them.
>
> ... I think the problem is often that people feel they haven't got time, they might die soon. Also they have, we all have been taught to accept things. Most people I see just want a practical solution to their problem ... if they can get that they are not going to take on the extra stress of court action. (Wilson, 1993, pp. 182–3)

If such views remain influential amongst advisors and those affected by HIV/AIDS they suggest that formal legal action is likely to occur only in a small minority of employment discrimination cases. Thus, even after the introduction of AIDS specific employment legislation a change in attitudes towards the usefulness of law may be required. Wilson's (1993) study shows that where a client received advice from a lawyer it was often possible to resolve the dispute without taking the case to court:

Many (lawyers) indicated that writing letters to landlords or employers threatening legal action often brought about a speedy out-of-court settlement which gave the client much needed financial compensation while at the same time saving them from the stress and trauma of a publicly fought dispute. (Wilson, 1993, p. 183)

As welcome to the aggrieved individuals as the compensation may be, it can be argued that there remains a need for legislation to produce an employment environment which is free from discriminatory practices against those with HIV/AIDS. The extent to which this is ever likely to be possible in practice, however, is open to question and has a number of parallels with attempts to outlaw sex and race discrimination (see, below), but whether or not specific AIDS employment law will achieve this objective, at this stage, remains to be seen. But to return to the examination of the existing legal provisions, one aspect of employment law on which both common law and more recent statutory legislation have a bearing is that of testing either prospective or existing employees for HIV.

Testing as Part of the Recruitment Procedure

There is no legal restriction which prevents employers requiring potential employees to submit to an HIV test as part of a pre-employment health check, and to refuse employment if the test is positive. However, since the taking of blood is not a routine procedure the doctor administering the HIV test will require the express consent of the applicant. This means that the doctor has to provide advice to the person so that they are able to make an informed choice as to whether to consent to the test (Harris and Haigh, 1990). In addition, it has been argued by Wilson (1992) that the test result is the property of the applicant and thus an employer would not be entitled to receive the result unless the applicant has given permission for its disclosure. However, since employers are not required to give *any* reason for their decision to refuse employment these provisions may be of limited value to prospective employees. A refusal either to take the test or to allow the results to be given to the employer may simply result in the applicant not being offered a job and having no form of legal redress.

An employer's right to reject an application for employment on any grounds, based upon a legal decision established in the last century (Allen v. Flood, 1898), is now constrained by more recent legislation outlawing discrimination on specific grounds, most notably sex (the Sex Discrimination Act, 1975 [SDA]) and race (the Race Relations Act, 1976 [RRA]). The former makes discrimination unlawful if decisions are made which can be shown to be based upon sex or marriage while the latter covers discrimination on the grounds of race, colour, nationality (including citizenship) or ethnic or national origins. Both these acts contain similar provisions dealing with direct and indirect discrimination and it has been argued that these provisions may be applicable to cases of recruitment testing of HIV status (Southam and Howard, 1988; Harris, 1990).

Thus, direct discrimination occurs where a person of one sex or racial group is treated less favourably on the ground of his/her sex or racial group than a person of the opposite sex or another racial group has been treated. In the context of HIV testing and an employer's requirement that applicants should test negative, the likelihood of succeeding with a claim under this legislation would depend upon the 'comparator' chosen (Wilson, 1992). For example, a gay man might succeed in such a claim if the tribunal allowed a lesbian as a comparator since currently more gay men than lesbians are HIV positive.

Indirect discrimination exists where a requirement or condition is applied to all employees (or prospective employees) but that a smaller proportion of one sex or racial group can comply. It is not necessary to show that there was an intention by the employer to discriminate; the motives of the discriminator are irrelevant: 'It is not a question of allocating blame, but of identifying the discriminatory consequences of particular actions and policies' (Gregory, 1987, p. 35). Thus the imposition of the requirement that prospective applicants for a job should be HIV negative could amount to unlawful indirect discrimination since, as a result of earlier transmission routes, current levels of infection are higher in men — in 1992 of the reported cases of AIDS only 13 per cent were women (IDS 1992) — and Africans, and these groups would be less able to comply with the requirement than would a woman or non-African applicant (Harris, 1990). But such a case would depend upon an examination of the statistical basis of HIV infection and the figures could vary significantly depending upon the area of the labour market from which potential employees are drawn.

Although the possibility of cases being brought under antidiscrimination law remains a possibility, at least while the level of HIV infection remains skewed in terms of gender and race, to date, no cases have been brought before a tribunal. However, the action of the Equal Opportunities Commission (EOC), whose functions include the elimination of discrimination on the ground of sex, in the 1987 case of the former airline Dan Air (noted in Chapter 2 above) is instructive of the possibilities that this legislation holds (EOC, 1987). Dan Air had an employment policy of recruiting only women for cabin crew posts. This policy had been in existence for thirty years and although the Company received sufficient unsolicited application to make the advertising of vacancies unnecessary, careers talks were only given to school*girls*; no man had ever been interviewed and there was evidence that men were discouraged from applying and a separate department within the company handled applications from male candidates. In its defence of the policy, Dan Air argued that their company doctor had advised against changing its policy until the diagnosis and treatment of AIDS became clearer and therefore that it had a defence under the 1974 Health and Safety at Work Act which required it to ensure the health and safety of employees and others who might be exposed to risk. The company supported their case by arguing that as HIV is principally transmitted by sexual intercourse, mainly affects homosexuals, that cabin staff are sexually promiscuous and that some 30 per cent of men who apply for cabin crew jobs are gay, then there was therefore a risk of transmission through blood and saliva to or from passengers if cabin staff cut themselves or if passengers required mouth-to-mouth resuscitation. The EOC, though, took expert medical opinion which suggested that there was no health risk to passengers provided that normal hygiene practice was followed. As a result of this investigation, the EOC issued a non-discrimination notice against Dan Air requiring it to change its recruitment practice and to produce evidence to show that this had been done. Thus, Southam and Howard (1988) conclude:

It is clear from this case that an employer who concludes that men are more likely to contract AIDS and should not, therefore, be recruited face a finding of unlawful discrimination under SDA 1975. (Southam and Howard 1988, p. 49)

Testing Existing Employees

In the case where an employer requires existing employees to take an HIV test, similar conditions to those outlined above pertain, that is, consent for the test and its disclosure to the employer. However, among the common law terms imported into every contract of employment is an implied duty of mutual trust and confidence and an employer must not act in a way which undermines this trust. In Bliss v South East Thames Regional Health Authority (a non-AIDS case of 1987) the court held that an employer who requires an employee to undergo a medical examination may be in breach of this duty. Unless, therefore, there is an express term written into the contract which allows for HIV testing then such a requirement by an employer might amount to a fundamental breach of the contract, allowing the employee to resign and, subject to having two years continuous service with the employer, be able to claim constructive unfair dismissal. There may be an exception to this general rule where the employee's job requires him/her to travel overseas and the country to which the employee is travelling demands a negative HIV test before granting entry.

In a recent example illustrating the application of this aspect of employment law, blood samples were taken from 132 catering staff at Harrods' food hall following an outbreak of food poisoning (Dodd and Nelson, 1994). Although the doctor was quoted as saying that the tests had been carried out as part of a wider health programme and that tests were made on the samples so that employees could receive treatment for a range of illnesses including diabetes, the samples were also tested for HIV. The newspaper article alleged that three of the tests were made on the employees after they had refused consent for HIV screening and were therefore illegal, while the remaining 129 might also be unlawful since these employees had not given express consent to HIV testing. In reviewing the employment law applicable to this case, Wilson (1994) argues that as far as HIV testing of employees is concerned there is a need for specific consent even if a blood sample is taken for other purposes:

> It would seem therefore that law and government policy have produced a situation where the boundaries of consent to blood testing are defined not by the way in which blood is taken, but by the nature of the diagnostic tests to be carried out on it. (Wilson, 1994, p. 576)

Thus, although it is reported that one chef is launching a test case and another has resigned, the article claims that many workers were angry about the tests but did not complain because they were afraid they would be sacked. Such concern amongst employees reflects the limited help that employment law can provide, particularly in periods of high unemployment where alternative work may be difficult to secure.

Perhaps more significantly for employers and fellow employees concerned about working with HIV positive employees and who see testing as a means of reducing the risk while at work, is that it is now well established that it can take between three and six months from infection for a test to show positive. Thus, an applicant who tests negative may well be already infected. Unless employers are prepared to arrange regular testing programmes (and employees are willing to take part in such a plan) it would appear that testing has very little practical benefit.

HIV/AIDS and Dismissal

Employment law has provided full-time employees who have two years' continuous service with their employer with statutory protection against being unfairly dismissed. An employee who has been dismissed may take a claim to an industrial tribunal. The test applied by tribunals in cases brought before them is firstly whether the employer can show a fair reason for dismissing the employee and secondly whether, in the circumstance of the case, the employer acted reasonably in treating the reason as grounds for dismissal. There are five reasons which the Employment Protection (Consolidation) Act 1978 includes as fair grounds for dismissal: lack of capability; misconduct; redundancy; statutory bar; and some other substantial reason. The two which are most relevant to cases of HIV/AIDS are those related to the capability of the employee to undertake the duties of the job, including the health of the employee, and 'some other substantial reason' sufficient to justify the dismissal of the employee.

Dismissal related to capability is likely to be relevant to those cases where an employee has developed AIDS and his/her state of health has declined to the extent that he/she is absent from work because of sickness, involving either long or short periods of frequent absence. Exceptionally, an employee who is able to work but whose performance has declined because of the illness may also be dismissed. In all these cases, if the employee is unable to perform the duties required under the contract of employment the employer may fairly terminate the contract. Although to date there have been no AIDS-related industrial tribunal cases on these grounds, the Department of Employment guidelines on HIV/AIDS state that a person who has become ill as a result of AIDS should not be treated differently from someone suffering 'any other non-contagious life threatening illness' (DOE/ HSE, 1987). Thus while each case of ill-health is to be treated on its own merits the guidelines laid down by the Employment Appeals Tribunal (EAT) on sickness dismissals in the 1977 case of East Lindsey District Council v Daubney are relevant. Here, the EAT stated that in ill-health cases employers need to acquaint themselves with the true medical position by obtaining a report from the employee's doctor including, if necessary, a report from an independent medical specialist, and personally consulting with the employee since this may bring to light facts of which the employer would otherwise be unaware. Provided the employer follows this guidance then the dismissal is likely to be regarded as fair. Clearly this is only likely to be so in cases where the employee has developed AIDS-related illness since those that are HIV positive and asymptomatic are unlikely to need any significant absences from work, or to be unable to fulfil their job requirements purely as a result of infection.

However, implicit in the way in which the test of reasonableness is applied in these cases is a recognition of the business interests of the employer and that these should be balanced against, if not take priority over, the needs of the employee. Indeed, industrial tribunals are specifically required to take account of the size and administrative resources of the employer's undertaking so lessening the chances of an employee of a small organization succeeding with a claim of unfair dismissal. Such needs for those who have developed AIDS include, of course, a degree of security which follows from having paid employment, and the self-esteem which employment may provide.

The category of 'some other substantial reason' allows employers to dismiss for a reason which does not easily fit into one of the other four categories. It has been used by employers in non-HIV cases to justify dismissals where fellow employees or customers of the employer object to the continued presence of an employee, and there is no legal reason why this could not be used against an employee known, or believed to be HIV positive. However, where the objections of fellow employees are claimed to constitute harassment against another employee, employers are required to provide support for the 'victim' and to consider the possibility of relocation and/or, if appropriate, disciplinary action against those employees responsible for the harassment. There are grounds for believing, however, that tribunals may uphold as fair the dismissal of someone with, or suspected of having HIV/AIDS. In the case of customer pressure, for example, employers may be able to justify a dismissal as fair even if there is no evidence that the employer is prejudiced against the employee. These circumstances arose in the 1981 case of Saunders v Scottish National Camps. Mr Saunders was employed to undertake general maintenance work at a holiday camp catering for children, but when his homosexuality was 'discovered' he was dismissed since the director feared a loss of business if Saunders remained employed. The company successfully argued that while *they* had no difficulty in continuing to employ him, a substantial minority of parents incorrectly believed that homosexuals are inevitably pederasts and would therefore not send their children to the camp. It has been argued by Watt (1992) that this case has important implications if applied to incidents involving HIV/AIDS:

> where an employee is honestly identified as (i) likely to be seropositive for HIV, or (ii) seropositive for HIV, or (iii) suffering from AIDS, by a person external to the enterprise, upon whom the enterprise relies as a significant source of income, the employer would be acting fairly in dismissing him ... In Saunders it became clear that there was no need for the dismissed person to have been proved to have the undesirable characteristic – in the Saunders case that of paederasty – as a matter of fact. *Any fear that a person possesses the characteristic does not need to be well-founded, merely honestly held.* (Watt, 1992, p. 86, emphasis added)

If this line of reasoning is correct then it will not be necessary for employers to show that an employee is HIV positive or had developed AIDS, but only that there was a genuine belief that this was the case. Similarly, the way in which other employees' beliefs and attitudes towards an employee can influence an employer's action and be supported by tribunals was shown in Cormack v TNT Sealion Ltd, 1986. This case concerned the claim of Mr Cormack, a ship's cook, that he had been unfairly selected for redundancy. He argued that he would not have found himself in a redundancy situation if it had not been for the fact that he had been unreasonably transferred from another vessel in the company's fleet. A number of his colleagues on Cormack's previous ship had strongly objected to sailing with him for 'personal hygiene' reasons — the innuendo being that he was a homosexual and thus, a carrier of the HIV virus. Although the tribunal stated that a good employer should act promptly to allay all unfounded suspicions and that it was not entirely satisfactory to transfer an employee in the hope that complaints would not recur, they nevertheless held the selection for redundancy to be fair. They went on to argue that Cormack's ability to fit in with his colleagues *was* a material fact for consideration in the selection process because of the particular kind of employment, that is, that ships' crews are required to live and work in close proximity. The implication of this case is that just as external pressure from customers may substantiate dismissal internal pressure from fellow employees can also provide sufficient justification for an employer to dismiss and for that dismissal to be found fair by an industrial tribunal. As one barrister has stated:

> ... if the employer does his best to reassure other employees, and their prejudice still ensures an unsatisfactory working environment, an industrial tribunal would be likely to find that a dismissal of an AIDS carrier [*sic*] was fair. (cited in IDS, 1987, p. 1)

However, there is evidence to suggest that tribunals will not always accept peer pressure as justification for dismissal. Indeed, there are cases where tribunals have upheld as fair the dismissal of the discriminators. The way in which tribunals will support employers who take action against the perpetrators rather than the victim of harassment was shown in Philpott v North Lambeth Law Centre 1986. In this case, a tribunal found the dismissal of two solicitors fair because of their attitude and behaviour towards a newly appointed solicitor at the law centre, Mr Haran, who prior to joining the organization had undertaken voluntary work for the Gay Switchboard. One of the two dismissed employees stated that his health was at risk as a result of Haran's appointment and requested Haran be required to work from home; the other complained to the Centre's health and safety officer and stated:

> Have you heard that they have appointed someone who will

introduce AIDS into the law centre? He has been working with Gay Switchboard. He could be infected. You should write to him and tell him not to come to the law centre. My family will hold you responsible if anything happens to me. (Quoted in Southam and Howard, 1988, p. 119–120)

The tribunal upheld the dismissals as being fair for, among other things, the malicious way the applicants had reacted to Mr Haran. However, from the AIDS-related cases reported, this approach does not seem to be typical of the courts' reasoning, and thus those employees who are HIV positive are more likely to be the ones losing their jobs than the perpetrators of discrimination.

The Limitations of Existing Law

The apparent inability of existing employment law to counteract cases of HIV discrimination is complicated by a number of features associated with the epidemic, not least of which is the element of moral panic that has accompanied the disease. Although the intensity of this panic has now diminished, it has not disappeared. Indeed, HIV/AIDS continues to pose a substantively different set of problems from other life-threatening or terminal diseases, involving (as was suggested in previous chapters), complex layers of meaning, intimately connected with sexuality and morality, with which many people who think of themselves as 'normal' feel distinctly uncomfortable. This situation has been exacerbated by the very novelty of the disease, its sudden discovery and apparently incurable effects: new hazards, especially those for which there is no immediate remedy, generate significant levels of fear and anxiety which, in turn, fuel perceptions of risk (Sim, 1992; Adam-Smith and Goss, 1993). In these respects, therefore, HIV/ AIDS is dissimilar to other serious diseases and its occurrence in workplace situations gives rise to questions which go well beyond those posed by other illnesses. In particular, the condition continues to be seen to be the result of what many regard as morally questionable behaviour. The extent to which HIV positive status is regarded as a correlate of homosexuality is indicated in the Swiss Institute for Comparative Law study (1993) which reports that the National Computer System of the British Police Force contains details of those 'suspected' of being HIV positive, a suspicion that is based on membership of a supposed 'risk group', as a result of which 'known' homosexuals are usually automatically listed as being HIV positive.

In the Cormack and Philpott cases reviewed above, the pressure placed upon employers to dismiss was closely related to the link made by work colleagues between HIV/AIDS and homosexuality. Further evidence of the impact of such a linkage emerges from the 1987 case of Buck v. Letchworth Palace Ltd. where it appeared to be a material factor in the minds of the tribunal in deciding that Mr Buck was not unfairly dismissed, their decision echoing the concerns summarised by Watt (1992) in the Saunders case (above). Here, Mr Buck had been employed as a cinema projectionist for 17 years but, following a report in a local newspaper that he had been convicted of gross indecency in a public toilet at Oxford Circus, two assistant projectionists refused to work with him. This, despite the fact that both they and the employer knew of Buck's earlier conviction for a similar offence in the early 1970s, led the co-workers to claim that they now feared that their shared toilet facilities might become contaminated with the 'AIDS virus'. As one of them said in a letter to the employer: '[We] feel that in view of the recent court case ... and knowing of his tendencies towards the male person, wish to state that we no longer care to work alongside or in the same proximity as Mr Buck' (cited in Watt, 1992, p. 88). Buck was subsequently sacked while on holiday and received a letter to this effect from the employer's solicitors stating that the decision to dismiss was taken as a result of his conviction and the fact that other projectionists were not prepared to continue working with him 'bearing in mind the increased public awareness of the AIDS epidemic and their general dislike of this sort of behaviour'. Although critical of the way in which the employer had handled the case, and recognizing that the objecting staff had overreacted, the tribunal nevertheless found the dismissal fair primarily on the grounds of Buck's acts of indecency. At no stage during the tribunal hearing was any evidence offered to prove that Mr. Buck had AIDS or was HIV positive. However, at the hearing the industrial tribunal went on to make clear that the linkage between homosexuality and AIDS justified his colleagues' response:

> they [the assistant projectionists] did nevertheless have genu-
> ine feelings which had been prompted by the applicant's
> offence in a public lavatory following his previous offence
> about which they knew, though which at the time did not cause

them undue concern. The publicity about AIDS had altered their reaction to the second offence, and we do not think it unreasonable that the respondents should have taken notice of this change. (cited in Watt, 1992, p. 87)

The outcome of this case can be cast along side one with essentially similar facts but where a tribunal came to a different conclusion. In Bell v Devon and Cornwall Police Authority (1978), Mr Bell was dismissed from his position as a chef at a police canteen following complaints from both civilian and police staff that they would refuse to eat in the canteen if Mr Bell remained in his post. Prior to his employment, Mr Bell had been arrested for two acts of gross indecency in a public toilet. He admitted at the magistrates court that he was bisexual but the prosecution failed and Mr Bell was found not guilty. The later industrial tribunal hearing of 1978 considered that the decision to dismiss Bell was based upon statements by staff that they would not eat food prepared by a homosexual and that the employer had not investigated the strength of the objections nor attempted to solve the problem by consultation and communication and, therefore, found the dismissal unfair. Although the Bell case occurred in 1978 well before AIDS became an issue, it remains illustrative of the fears and prejudices to which, in this case, homosexuality can give rise, especially in areas commonly perceived to be sites of potential 'infection' such as medical care or food preparation (see, Armstrong 1983; Lupton, 1994b). Indeed, it seems that 'otherness' itself all too easily corresponds to 'threat', including threat of (actual and symbolic) infection, and when this can be linked, however misguidedly, with a real viral agent, the potential for discrimination is clearly magnified.

These cases also raise another important issue in relation to HIV/AIDS, however, namely confidentiality. The law relating to confidentiality is also open to different interpretation. According to Gaymer 1989:

The duty of trust and confidence in the employment relationship requires that the employer and employee should keep information on the HIV status of any employee confidential unless the employee consents to disclosure. Disclosure without consent may however be justified in the public interest in very exceptional cases if, for example, there is a threat to the health and safety of others. (Gaymer, 1989, p. 1)

In relation to the 'public interest' issue, the 1988 case of X vs Y indicates that this is a highly constrained possibility. The court ruled that it was not in the public interest for a national newspaper to reveal medical records which showed that two general practitioners had AIDS and were continuing to practice. It was shown that 'any risk posed by the doctors was theoretical and would be eliminated if they had the confidence to report the diagnosis to their employer' (Harris, op cit, p. 91).

Disclosure without consent will usually only be justified to those needing to know, such as a first aider. Gaymer also suggests that in the absence of an express contractual term, a person with HIV/AIDS is not under an obligation to reveal this to an employer except where not to do so would lead to the risk of infection or harm to others, breaching the employee's statutory obligation under section 7 of the HSAW 1974. Again, and in line with the advice given in the government's *AIDS and the Workplace*, such risks are, for most people, negligible. Clearly, the maintenance of confidentiality raises a number of practical problems ranging from the operation of the 'rumour mill' to the pressuring of an individual to divulge a confidence. In the latter case, it is of some concern to note an apparent increase in the cases of pressure being placed on occupational health nurses by personnel managers to reveal details of employees' medical records (*Personnel Management Plus*, 1994). Such disclosure would, of course, not only be of dubious legality but could also result in a nurse being 'struck off' (see also Lesslie, 1994).

Conclusion

The material we have presented in this chapter suggests that as current British employment law stands those with HIV/AIDS enjoy limited protection from discrimination. As Wilson (1994) points out, the thrust of legislation in Britain has been rather to protect 'healthy citizens': 'From the perspective of the so-called "general public" the law has been very protective. Protecting the majority of the (supposedly) uninfected from the minority of the known infected population' (Wilson, 1994, p. 17). The few cases concerning HIV/AIDS that have reached the employment courts seem, in general, to support this view that protection is afforded to those who perceive themselves to be at risk from a supposedly infected 'other', even if there is little or no evidence that the 'other' is HIV positive.

The key difficulty lies, perhaps, in the way in which discrimination is socially conceived and acted upon: a problem that legal measures may not be the most effective instrument to overcome. To this extent, there are clear similarities with causes of discrimination on the grounds of race and sex to which many writers have drawn attention (Atkins and Hoggert, 1984; Cockburn, 1991; Gregory and O'Donovan, 1985; Fitzpatrick, 1987). Although the history of AIDS is too short to have developed a deep seated prejudice that is characteristic of sexism and racism many of the components for such a development exist, particularly as a result of its link with homosexuality.

Thus, although typically referred to as providing 'rights' for employees, Anderman (1992) argues that British employment protection law may be more appropriately viewed as a form of regulation of management decisions.

From this perspective the emphasis is placed on the way legislative rules . . . operate to strike a balance between workers' rights and another value — the value of managerial autonomy to make decisions. This is useful to highlight the way legislation as drafted often invites a regulatory line to be drawn by industrial tribunals or judges which is not necessarily in accord with the values of Parliament. (Anderman, 1992, p. v)

A characteristic feature of the courts' approach in striking this balance is that in judging management decisions, account has to be taken of what it is 'reasonable' to expect an employer to decide in a particular case. Rather than talk of an employee's 'right not to be unfairly dismissed' it may be more precise to regard this as a right not to be *unreasonably* dismissed since the assessment of unfairness must take account of what the court believes to be reasonable action by the employer. Thus, the protection provided by statute is rarely absolute for employees: it is qualified by the recognition by the legislators that an employer must be allowed to conduct the business in the most efficient manner, subject only to the limited requirements imposed by legislation. It is perhaps for this reason that no matter how grossly unfairly an employee is dismissed the tribunals have no power to force an employer to reinstate the worker: they are limited only to enhancing the employee's compensation if an employer refuses to comply with a decision to reinstate. Indeed, it can be argued that in many employment cases, all the law has done is to place a financial penalty on employers for a failure to accept the requirements of legal regulation of their decisions. In a survey of dismissed employees who claimed re-employment at an industrial tribunal Lewis (1981) discovered that only 72 per cent of respondents claimed this remedy and that this had dropped to 20 per cent by the time of the hearing. Further, of those who continued to claim 're-employment' only 57 per cent of these obtained such an order and in almost two-thirds of these the employer refused to abide by the order.

It would appear, therefore, that unless specific legislation is introduced which provides a positive assertion of non-discrimination coupled with effective remedies, then the position of those with HIV/ AIDS in employment is likely to depend upon whether employers see the law as a constraint on their freedom to manage which is to be minimized or as a basis for the constructive development of policies and practices towards those affected. Whether such law is likely to be forthcoming will in part depend on whether a sufficiently strong lobby for its introduction can be developed and maintained. This in itself may be supported by legal developments in other countries and it is to legal developments outside Britain that the next chapter is devoted.

Chapter 7

Legislative Responses to HIV/AIDS in Europe and the USA

Introduction

The relationship between the various elements of British employment law and the cases of those employees who are HIV positive or have developed AIDS has been explored in the previous chapter. It was suggested that the law's coverage is significantly incomplete, with the result that it does not necessarily provide the basis for the positive encouragement of constructive organizational responses, and provides a highly uncertain degree of protection to affected employees. In concluding this investigation of the legislative responses to HIV/AIDS, this chapter considers the legal approaches to the issue taken in Europe and the United States of America. The latter is especially significant because of the treatment of people with HIV/AIDS within the Americans With Disabilities Act (ADA), although measures originating in the European Union may also have implications for cases where detriment results from an employer or other employees assuming a causal link between HIV infection and homosexuality.

European Legislation

It is beyond the scope of this chapter to provide a detailed examination of national laws; rather the purpose is to expose similarities and differences in the application of the law. The general picture that emerges from a review of employment legislation in other European countries is one that is broadly similar to British experience. No country has introduced specific employment law dealing with people who are HIV positive or who have developed AIDS and, thus, employers have considerable freedom to develop their own response. Similarly, employees who feel they have suffered discrimination because of their infection have to rely upon the provisions of existing employment law. The situation has been summarized in a wide ranging study of employment law and AIDS by the Swiss Institute of Comparative Law thus:

> European countries' labour legislation has not been modified to deal with this epidemic. It is therefore for the courts to establish principles by interpreting the existing law when cases are brought before them. But the whole difficulty arises from the fact that those who are HIV-positive or suffer from AIDS very often refrain from bringing a judicial action for physical, psychological, financial or social reasons. This explains the paucity of case law on the subject. (Swiss Institute, 1993, p. 124)

This view is clearly identifiable with the British position examined in Chapter 6. However, on some particular issues related to AIDS significant differences exist which are worthy of note.

The general tendency in other European countries is not to provide for the routine HIV screening as far as employment is concerned, an approach that is consistent with British practice. While UK law does not forbid an HIV test at the recruitment stage, the legal system in other European countries contain alternative and more prohibitive provisions. In Italy, the Constitution specifically prohibits both public and private employers from carrying out tests to establish possible HIV infection in both current and prospective employees, and any breach of the law makes the employer subject to prosecution. Italian law also extends protection to those with HIV or AIDS by making the transfer of an employee on these grounds unlawful, even if its purpose is to protect other employees (Swiss Institute, 1993). The Catalonian Parliament in Spain has passed a resolution which has the effect of outlawing discrimination against infected people at the recruitment stage (Rieben Schizas, 1995). Similarly, in forbidding any discrimination based upon race, religion, sex, political opinions or any other grounds, the Constitution of the Netherlands implies a general prohibition of discrimination on grounds of health, thereby making compulsory HIV testing unlawful (Swiss Institute, 1993).

As far as refusal of employment on the grounds of HIV infection is concerned legislation in other European countries is broadly similar to that in Britain. Such a refusal is usually lawful provided there is no discrimination on the grounds of sex, race, disability or on other specific grounds covered by existing legal measures. Most countries recognize that 'fitness for the job' is a major employment criterion and, as such, people who have developed AIDS may find employment difficult to obtain and, incidentally, have little protection against dismissal. However, employment law in Sweden gives the employer the specific right to refuse employment to an HIV-positive applicant and the airline, SAS, operates such a policy. In addition, Swedish law considers that the employer has the right to include in an employee's contract the obligation to undergo regular screening examinations (Westerhall and Saldeen, 1992, p. 36).

Like Britain, no European country allows for dismissal of employees solely on the grounds of being HIV positive. In general, the lawfulness or otherwise of a dismissal depends upon the construction of the law in each country regulating an employer's ability to dismiss an employee, although the standard of protection provided by employment law varies between countries. For example, Belgian employment law allows a contract of employment to be terminated at the employer's discretion and the employer is not required to give a reason for the dismissal. However, in the Netherlands an employer wishing to dismiss an employee must obtain the authorization of the Regional Employment Directorate and this body has refused to permit the dismissal of an HIV positive hospital worker who had been absent for three months on sick leave. Where an HIV positive employee is dismissed because of the pressure other employees (a situation which the previous chapter has shown to have occurred in Britain) a German court has decided that the provision of information to deal with the irrational fears of work colleagues is a responsibility of the employer (Rieben Schizas, 1995).

Characteristically, therefore, legal protection for those with HIV/AIDS in the wider European employment context is broadly similar to that in Britain, in that no country has developed wholly specific legislation related to the employment aspects of the epidemic, relying instead on existing or amended employment legislation. Only where this established legislation is more constraining on management decisions (for example, as regards dismissal in the Netherlands) are employees affected by HIV likely to find greater protection. In general, then, those who have developed AIDS will be subject to the provisions relating to a dismissal on the grounds of ill-health. That is, a dismissal for sickness reasons will depend for its fairness on the circumstances of the case, for example, the length or regularity of absence from work, the prognosis of the individual employee's illness, possibilities of redeployment, the need to replace the employee because of the position held within the organization and the extent to which the employee's absence has a negative impact upon the employer's business. The legal protection provided to HIV positive employees or those with AIDS is generally, therefore, a function of the level of protection afforded to any employee against unfair dismissal.

A possible exception to this trend is to be found in France where recent legislation potentially provides for a greater level of regulation concerning the treatment of employees who are HIV positive and, possibly, for those who have developed AIDS. Measures passed in 1990 have aimed at making unlawful any discrimination on the grounds of an individual's state of health or disability, including discrimination related to seropositivity. Refusal of employment or dismissal on these grounds is punishable by imprisonment and/or a fine except (mirroring other aspects of employment law) in cases where fitness for employment is medically certified. In addition, the legislation contains measures which would seem to help in those cases where the potential for stress or publicity may deter those affected taking a claim to court. Under these provisions HIV/AIDS support groups are able to take legal proceedings on behalf of those who feel they have suffered from discrimination (Rieben Schizas, 1995). Indeed, the principle of including HIV/AIDS within a law designed to offer protection to those with disabilities has similarities with the Americans With Disabilities Act which is examined below. Before this, we turn to a consideration of the relevance to those with HIV/AIDS of European Union measures.

European Union Measures

The focus of the European Union (and its predecessor the European Community) has been on the public health aspects of AIDS through, for example, the Europe Against AIDS Programme, an approach echoed in Britain, rather more notoriously, in the 'Tombstones and Icebergs' publicity campaign (Berridge, 1992). However, as was noted in chapter 1, in 1989 the Council of Ministers for Health did adopt a wide-ranging resolution, the Fight Against AIDS, which in employment terms recommended that, 'The greatest possible vigilance must therefore be exercised in order to combat all forms of discrimination in recruitment, at the workplace ... and sickness insurance (*Social Europe*, 1990, p. 156). Perhaps more significantly, Britain's membership of the European Union (EU) has meant that it has now to implement legislation required of it as part of the conditions of membership. Typically this means passing new or amending existing laws to meet the requirements of EU Directives. In addition, EU Recommendations, while not regarded as legally binding, may also play an important role as 'national courts are bound to take them into account when deciding disputes before them where that Recommendation clarifies the interpretation of national provisions enacted to implement it or where the Commission intended the Recommendation to supplement binding Community measures' (IDS, 1993b, p. 148).

It is possible, therefore, that the application of one Recommendation of the EU may have significance in the context of HIV/AIDS where an employee suffers a detriment (dismissal, or merely put under a disadvantage) and the underlying reason for this is the person's perceived sexual orientation. In the 1993 case of Wadham v Carpenter Farrer Partnership, the British Employment Appeals Tribunal (EAT) stated that tribunals may derive assistance from the EU Recommendation and Code of Practice on the Dignity of Women and Men at Work (EU, 1991). These provisions, adopted following a European Community Council Resolution the previous year, deal with sexual harassment at work, defining it as: '... unwanted conduct of a sexual nature, or other conduct based on sex affecting the dignity of women and men at work (EU, 1991, pp. 49/4). Article 1 of the Recommendation states that such conduct will be unacceptable if it is unwanted, unreasonable and offensive to the recipient, or rejection or submission to such conduct is used as a basis for a decision which affects job opportunities, continued employment, promotion, salary or any other employment decisions, or creates an intimidating, hostile or humiliating work environment for the recipient. The Employment Appeal Tribunal suggested that these clauses may help in determining whether an employee had suffered a 'detriment' in sex discrimination cases. The Code goes on to list specific groups, particularly vulnerable to sexual harassment, including lesbians and gay men, thereby bringing sexual orientation within the scope of sexual harassment:

It is undeniable that harassment on the grounds of sexual

orientation undermines the dignity at work of those affected and it is impossible to regard such harassment as appropriate workplace behaviour. (EU, 1991, p. 49/3)

Tribunals in the cases of Buck (examined in Chapter 6 above) and other similar claims have stated that if the dismissal was solely on the grounds of others objecting to working with the ex-employee on the grounds of his homosexuality *per se*, then they may well have been considered unfair. However, further support for discrimination on grounds of sexual orientation being unlawful and thus confirming the relevance of the EU Code comes from a recent industrial tribunal case. In the 1993 case of Wallace & O'Rouke v BG Turkey Services (Scotland) Ltd, the two female applicants alleged that they were dismissed by the respondent because they were having a lesbian relationship with each other. They argued that since a man would not have been dismissed if he had formed a relationship with a female worker then their dismissal must have been based upon their gender and was thus unlawful direct discrimination under the Sex Discrimination Act 1975 (SDA). Although the case was settled before a full hearing was held, the tribunal in its preliminary hearing indicated that an employer's action against an employee on the grounds of the person's sexuality or sexual preferences can amount to discrimination under the Act. Clearly this case cannot be taken as a firm statement of the law, but as Bamforth (1994) suggests:

... this interpretation of (the SDA), if correct, offers a greater degree of protection to persons of non-heterosexual orientation than has previously been offered in English or Scottish law, and to that extent must be welcomed, given the widespread social hostility directed at such persons. (Bamforth, 1994, p. 1419)

The combination of the EU Recommendation and these developments in the application of British employment law hold out the possibility for greater employment protection for gay men and lesbians and may be relevant to cases where employees are discriminated against because of the perceived link between their sexual orientation and HIV.

USA Employment Legislation

The experience of the effects of HIV/AIDS on employment relations in the USA has resulted in greater development of both employment practice and employment law than is evident in the UK (Kelly, 1989, 1992; Kohl *et al*, 1990; Feldman, 1991). Although the decade of the 1980s was marked by declarations by most States that discrimination on the grounds of HIV/AIDS was wrong, only a few such as Florida and Iowa had backed up this stance with anti-discriminatory legislation. The result of this piecemeal approach was a lack of consistency in the application of law on discrimination, leading one commentator to conclude that the cause was due in part to '... the myriad of federal, state, local law and administrative regulations, as well as a considerable amount of judge made law' (Kelly, 1989, p. 502). What was needed, it was argued, was a federal response, a view emphasised by Admiral Watson, former Chairperson of the President's Commission on the HIV Epidemic. In his testimony to the Senate Committee on the Handicapped which was considering the introduction of wide ranging legislation aimed at prohibiting discrimination more generally on the grounds of disability he said:

> as long as discrimination occurs and no strong national policy with rapid and effective remedies against discrimination is established, individuals who are infected with HIV will be reluctant to come forward for testing, counselling and care. This fear of potential discrimination ... will undermine efforts to contain the epidemic and will leave HIV infected individuals isolated and alone. (ADA, 1990, p. 31)

As a result of these arguments, infection with HIV was covered by the provisions of the Americans With Disabilities Act, 1990 (ADA) and thus is similar to the aims of French law noted above. The ADA seeks to outlaw discrimination against those with disabilities in a number of areas including public services and transport. In the employment field, the Act specifies that an employer:

> shall not discriminate against a qualified individual with a disability in regard to job application procedures, the hiring, advancement, or discharge of employees, employee compensation, job training and other terms, conditions or privileges of

employment. (ADA, 1990, Section 102[a])

The Act also prevents an employer from 'limiting, segregating or classifying' job applicants or existing employees in such a way that employment opportunities or status are adversely affected.

Disability under the Act has a three-pronged definition and means an individual who has:

A) a physical or mental impairment that substantially limits one or more of the major life activities of such individual;
B) a record of such impairment: or
C) being regarded as having such an impairment. (ADA, 1990, Section 3[2]).

In addition to being noted as a specific disability within the scope of the Act, HIV/AIDS is covered by the first prong of the definition. A person infected with HIV, it is suggested, would have a substantial limitation of major life activities, i.e procreation and intimate sexual relationships; those who have developed AIDS would progressively suffer from a range of physiological disorders. Indeed, although the impossibility of producing a comprehensive list of all the conditions covered by the definition was noted in the Act, infection with HIV was specifically mentioned as being included as a disability.

The interpretation of the third prong of the definition provides some possibility of protection where there is a link made between HIV infection and homosexuality. Despite some attempts to include same-gender sexual orientation within the Act (Lee and Brown, 1993), homosexuality is specifically excluded from its scope: Section 511 of the Act stating:

For the purposes of the definition of 'disability' ... homosexuality and bisexuality are not impairments and *as such* are not disabilities under this Act. (emphasis added) (ADA, 1990, Section 511)

In its discussion of the meaning of 'being regarded as having such an impairment' the Senate Committee drew attention to the possibility of a social construction of disability. It noted that society's accumulated myths and fears about disability and diseases can be as handicapping for the individual as the physical or mental limitations that flow from the impairment, and that this may be particularly relevant in the employment context:

> A person who is excluded from any basic life activity, or is otherwise discriminated against, because of [an employer's] negative attitude towards that impairment is treated as having a disability. Thus, for example, if an employer refuses to hire someone because of a fear of the 'negative reactions' of others to the individual or because of the employer's perception that the applicant has an impairment which prevents that person from working that person is covered under the third prong of the definition of disability. (ADA, 1990, p. 53)

Although particularly concerned with stigmatic conditions, for example severe burns, that are viewed as physical impairments but do not in fact result in any major limitation of life activity, this element of the definition may provide some degree of legal protection for gay men who are refused employment because of the belief of employers, and existing employees, that they are, or are more likely to be, HIV positive. The success of such cases would presumably rest on an individual's ability to persuade a court that, say, a job offer was denied, not because of the applicant's sexual orientation *as such* but because of the connection made between it and the greater likelihood of HIV infection. Whether this interpretation of the legislation is accepted will have to await the outcome of a test case in the American courts. Its importance may have significance, however, in the light of attempts to introduce similar legislation in Britain discussed in the previous chapter and the similarity in definition used.

Where an employee or applicant for an employment position with such an impairment is able to perform the essential functions of the job then the person is regarded as a 'qualified individual' and an employer must make 'reasonable accommodation' for the person. This may involve taking steps to ensure existing facilities are accessible and usable and/or other measures including, say, job restructuring, part-time work and transfer to more appropriate work. Such accommodation is required of employers only when they are aware of a person's disability. While the Act envisages times when an employer may become aware that an employee is having difficulty performing a task and may therefore discuss the possibility of help, it is expected that the employer's duty to accommodate is likely to be triggered by a request from an applicant or employee (ADA, 1990, p. 65). In what may be seen as an attempt to protect the privacy of an employee and to maintain confidentiality in the employment relationship it would appear that making accommodation without such a request (or without an employee's agreement) would be unlawful, particularly if such accommodation has an adverse affect on the individual. This could be the case if changes were made to an employee's duties without consent and fellow employees behaved prejudicially towards the employee believing the changes made to be the result of HIV infection. One example from American case law illustrates this point. In Chalk v. US District Court (1988), the Circuit Court decided that it was unlawful unilaterally to transfer to an administrative post a teacher supposedly 'handicapped' (*sic*) by HIV because the overwhelming weight of medical evidence was that social contact between the teacher and children posed no significant risk of transmission (Kelly, 1989). The principles underlying this decision seem to bear close resemblance to those made in the Equal Opportunities Commission's investigation of Dan Air's practice of only employing women cabin staff (see, chapter 6 above).

Furthermore, an employer may not require a disabled applicant to undergo a medical examination related to the disability unless the examination is required of *all* applicants. Similarly, an employer is prohibited from requiring medical examinations of existing employees 'unless such examination or inquiry is shown to be job-related and consistent with business necessity' (ADA, 1990, Section 102 (c) 4 (B)). This clause, if applied to Britain, would clearly strengthen the existing provisions on testing examined above.

The Act thus seeks to eliminate employment discrimination against those with disabilities by laying down three key requirements: individuals with disabilities are not rejected because of their inability to perform non-essential or marginal job functions, selection criteria that screen out those with disabilities may only be applied if they are job related and consistent with business necessity and, for both applicants and existing employees, reasonable accommodation at work is made where necessary. In their summary of the position of people with disabilities the Committee commented as follows:

> The unfortunate truth is that individuals with disabilities are a discrete, specific minority who have been insulated in many respects from the general public. Such individuals have been faced with a range of restrictions and limitations in their lives.

Further they have been subjected to unequal and discriminatory treatment in a range of areas, based on characteristics that are beyond the control of such individuals and resulting from stereotypical assumptions, fear and myths not truly indicative of the ability of such individuals to participate in and contribute to society. Finally, such individuals have often not had the political power and muscle to demand the protections that are rightly theirs. (ADA, 1990, p. 40)

Although referring to those with disabilities in general, these remarks have clear application for those with HIV/AIDS particularly in relation to stereotypes, myths and fear. In addition, the Act also outlaws discrimination by an employer (by excluding or otherwise denying access to equal jobs or benefits) against an individual who has a relationship or association with a person who has a known disability. This protection is not limited to those who have a familial relationship with the disabled individual and it would appear that, in the context of HIV/AIDS, this would prohibit employment discrimination against a person caring for, or living with, someone with HIV/AIDS. Certainly, the possibility of 'discrimination by association' in the context of HIV/AIDS was made known to the Committee in testimony concerning a long serving female employee who was dismissed from her job when her employer discovered that her son, who had become ill with AIDS, had moved into her house so she could care for him (ADA, 1990, p. 30). However, the protection afforded by this provision appears to be limited in that an employer is not required to make any accommodation for the non-disabled employee. Thus, if the employee breaks a 'disabled-neutral' employer policy concerning, for example, attendance, he or she may be dismissed even if the reason for the absence was to care for the disabled person.

Conclusions

The ADA has only been operational since 1992 and it is thus too early to draw any conclusions concerning its effectiveness particularly as far as discrimination on the grounds of HIV/AIDS is concerned. Like all legislation its success in meeting its objectives will depend to a large extent on the interpretation the courts take of its provisions. However, in producing an Act with the purpose of providing 'a clear and comprehensive national mandate for the elimination of discrimination against individuals with disabilities' and the provision of 'clear, strong, consistent enforceable standards addressing discrimination against individuals with disabilities' (ADA, 1990, section 2(b)) the legislature has provided a clear benchmark against which the actions of employers can be judged.

However, despite the apparent adoption of key components of the wording of this act in the emerging disability legislation in the UK, there may be little grounds for real optimism in this regard. The Conservative government's approach to this issue has been carefully to avoid treading a path that offers positive rights to disadvantaged groups, favouring instead to provide limited and conditional protections from further mistreatment. Ultimately, what is at stake here is not the wording of specific pieces of legislation but the wider issue of the general culture of citizenship and civil rights within which these are activated and, in this respect, it is not entirely surprising that most progress seems to have been made in America and France where these notions are relatively well established. Thus, it seems that the fight against discrimination and prejudice towards those affected by HIV/AIDS cannot be fought on the battlefield of detailed legislation alone, but must also address the questions of citizenship rights on a more general level. As will be discussed in the following chapter, while it must be accepted that HIV/AIDS raises its own unique problems, especially within employing organizations, these cannot necessarily be remedied through single-issue campaigns and policies.

Chapter 8

Conclusions

The spread of the HIV epidemic has posed numerous problems for employing organizations. Even though the number of infected employees and the consequent loss of human resources in the western industrial countries has not been as great as was anticipated early in the epidemic, the HIV virus has left its imprint on many aspects of organizational practice. On the one hand, there are the lives that have been disrupted and damaged by prejudicial and discriminatory practices but, on the other hand, there have also been attempts to improve, within the sphere of the workplace, the understanding of difference and to develop a more just and tolerant practice. In effect, the epidemic has served to expose many of the principles of organization that are normally taken as given and, in particular, it has revealed operations of power and control that are frequently submerged in the ebb and flow of 'ordinary organizational life'. Thus, the epidemic has threatened a potential disruption of the key organizing principle of rationality and what has been detailed in the preceding chapters can be read as attempts by actors, in various capacities and through various institutions, to achieve either a reorganization or a protection of these established principles.

In the case of most European employment law, for instance, the unwillingness of states to embark upon a legislative process that offers a positive right of non-discrimination to persons with HIV/AIDS can be seen as having the effect (intentional or otherwise) of protecting established interests within the socio-economic sphere. As Wilson (1994) points out:

> ... law would seem to legitimate the already existent hierarchies of power. In the case of HIV protection we see therefore law constructed on the basis of the existing hierarchy of the

(supposedly) uninfected over the infected. The HIV positive person thus becomes the 'other' over whom control is legitimate ... Secondly ... at the moment we have only abstract rights for people with HIV, rather than real or concrete rights. That is, the case law which would seem to grant a right of non-discrimination to a person affected (or believed to be affected) by HIV is framed in vague terms which leave much discretion to the powerful ... at present employment protection law is grounded in utilitarian principles; that is, in terms of what is good for a workforce in general. The good of the individual is decided on a case by case basis within a utilitarian framework of the greatest good of the greatest number. Thus, if the greatest number feel irrationally scared of working with someone who is HIV positive, then that person may lose his or her job. (Wilson, 1994, pp. 19–20)

This characteristic, which particularly applies to UK employment law, can clearly be seen to be mirrored in the logic of the defensive responses outlined in chapter 2, where the emphasis is firmly on the threat of harm to the established interests of the organization and its majority members, and the development of conditional and exclusionary policies to deal with those who are defined as representing such a threat. Wilson's alternative to this form of law is to advocate the consideration of an approach to HIV non-discrimination based on de-ontological principles, that is, the construction of the individual's rights in such a way that these rights exist 'irrespective of social utility', such that the law would then embrace a positive assertion of non-discrimination (1994, p. 20). In the same way that existing legal logics are reflected in defensive responses so, it can be argued, a de-ontological stance, perhaps of the sort embedded in the ADA, is implicit in constructive responses to the epidemic.

However, as was argued in chapter 3 there are also potential difficulties with this approach, not only in terms of reconciling it with wider cultural expectations that may be hostile to the extension of the citizenship/civil rights project. On the one hand, as Wilson (op cit) recognizes, is the necessity for this type of approach to make HIV/AIDS an ontological reality for the infected person, that is, a master-status within which other aspects of identity and being are subsumed, if not submerged. While this may be the price that has to be paid for effective legal protection it does pose problems of 'abnormalization' if AIDS retains its profile as an 'exceptional' condition, particularly so when the master status of 'dread disease' is used to reinforce prejudice against already stigmatized identities. On the other hand, whereas a strongly de-ontological stance could be seen to lead to a stigmatized separatism, the opposite extreme is normative assimilation, where the promise of fair treatment is conditional upon the denial not just of a stigmatized identity but *any* collective identification that does not conform to dominant notions of normality. Here, ironically, the desire to suppress the stigmatic effects of 'AIDS-association' may, simultaneously and perhaps unconsciously, also be an attempt to suppress those identities that have suffered from 'association': silencing the 'victims' for fear that their cries will awaken us to our own role in contributing to their calamity. As Patton (1990, p. 131) has remarked: 'The AIDS narrative exists as a technology of social repression; it is a representation that attempts to silence not only the claims of identity politics, but the people marginalized by AIDS'. Thus, in a paradoxical way the incidence of HIV and AIDS can readily bring to the surface the pervasive strands of homophobia and 'compulsory heterosexuality' that underlie much 'normal' organization, but it can also give rise to 'solutions' that reproduce and perpetuate these inequalities rather than challenging them. Ironically, these normalizing solutions may have the appearance of being progressive and humane, but their wider political impact may be to mirror the prejudices more openly expressed in crude defensive responses.

A similar effect is experienced in relation to illness. In most organizations there is a well understood distinction between sickness and health — an institutionalized 'sick-role' so to speak — with the transition between the two states generally being relatively unambiguous and unremarkable, that is to say, those who are accredited as medically sick 'leave' the organization until they are certified well or unable to continue work (see, Goss, 1994b). HIV makes this distinction problematic not only because of the way in which it evokes widespread fear of infection, thereby drawing disproportionate attention to the presence of the 'infected' within the organization, but also because of the inherently ambiguous nature of the viral infection. Thus, a person may be known to be infected but not be ill, although, as Sontag (1991) has pointed out, neither may they be regarded as wholly 'well'. This contradictory status raises questions about the nature of any concessions the organization should make to preserve an infected employee's health. As Cockburn (1991) has remarked in relation to the more general issue of disability:

> ... employers ... take a blinkered view of their responsibility for
> disabled people. At best they wonder, 'Could this disabled person
> possibly do the job we are offering?' It is a rare employer who
> thinks 'Which jobs could we restructure ... to make it feasible for
> a person with this disability to do them?' Even less do employers
> evaluate the organization and its jobs by criteria of health. 'Are we
> a health promoting organization? Do we threaten the health of
> our employees?' (Cockburn, 1991, p. 206)

In addition, however, there is the widespread equation of HIV infection
with imminent death to contend with, and death is another subject that
unsettles many of the normal discourses of rational organization.
According to Bauman, death can be seen as 'the ultimate failure of
rationality': the human inability to reconcile the 'transcending power
of time-binding mind and the transience of its time-bound fleshy
casing' (cited in Mellor and Schilling, 1993, p. 412). For the individual
employee, too strong an engagement with matters of death threatens
normal processes of organization: it contaminates rational decision-
making with emotion (that is, grief, and often guilt; see James, 1993).
It undermines continuity of performance based on career and 'succes-
sion', it calls into question commitment to the organization as the key
facet of work identity: 'The uncertainty resulting from the certainty
[/possibility] of an early death invariably goes hand in hand with a new
evaluation of what was previously thought to be important and have
meaning' (Sievers, 1993, p. 19). In short, and in the absence of well
established institutional 'coping mechanisms' of the sort associated
with work that routinely deals with death, the individual's confrontation with death reframes organizational claims to continuity and,
simultaneously, the behaviours which reproduce it over time.

Indeed, this is not dissimilar to the effect which the discourse of
AIDS can have on the more general claims of rational organization. As
Weeks points out:

> ... we are living in a culture that at one time seemed to promise
> the triumph of technology over the uncontrollable whims of
> nature, and yet here is a new virus that has apparently
> confounded science ... 'The impact of aids is essentially linked
> to modernity — its virulence and relative untreatability lead us
> to question a cornerstone of faith in science, experts and
> progress'. (Weeks, 1991, p. 115)

This uncertainty can be seen in the emotional dilemmas to which HIV/AIDS gives rise within employment situations. At one level HIV/AIDS policies, especially written ones, can be seen as an attempt to reintroduce elements of rationality into responses, but in practice these are likely to remain largely at the level of abstract formality, often removed from the subjective understandings and emotional uncertainties that characterize both the direct experience of HIV/AIDS and the deep anxieties it arouses in others.

Thus, when HIV/AIDS is considered at the level of organizational policy it is most likely to be framed as a moral *issue* ('easy to name', acontextual, widely agreed upon, amenable to simple choice between 'right' and 'wrong'). At this level, organizations require the appearance of rationality and generality: clear and unified statements of purpose applicable to the organization as a totality, unambiguous and unequivocal. However, once an issue has been thus framed, it has then to be tested in practice. Organization actors have to use issue-based policy codes as guides to practical action in specific rather than general situations. They have to approach these codes not only as the agents of organizational interests, but also as unique individuals with their own personal morality and interests. It is at this level, the level of individual action, that a moral issue inscribed in a policy code will become a moral *dilemma*: hard to name, context-specific, contentious, complex and conflicting, not amenable to clear judgments. And in this regard the complex, emotional and messy reality of interpersonal relations seldom lends itself to the simple application of a priori policy prescriptions.

In all these ways, therefore, HIV and AIDS poses a challenge to the rational 'front' of most ordinary workplace organization. In particular, it threatens the 'official' identities that have been constructed for both individuals and organizations, by bridging the normally taken-for-granted boundaries between 'front-stage' and 'back-stage' presentations of self. Importantly, however, these challenges are multiple and dispersed. HIV and AIDS have not presented employing organizations in the west with the frontal attack of devastating proportions that was expected in the mid-1980s, and despite being a new medical condition, neither has it faced organizations with wholly new challenges. Rather it has activated and magnified existing inequalities, fears and prejudices: fear of the sick and dying; homophobia; racism; sexism. Thus, we would argue that for employing organizations, any adequate 'solution' to the workplace problems posed by HIV/AIDS will need to address these issues simultaneously. Without this 'long agenda' approach responses to HIV/AIDS in the workplace may be humane but they may also be less than human.

References

ABERCROMBIE, N. and WARDE, A. (1994) *Contemporary British Society*, Cambridge, Polity.

ADA (1990) *The Americans with Disabilities Act of 1990*, 101st Congress.

ADAM-SMITH, D. and GOSS, D. (1993) 'HIV/AIDS and hotel and catering employment: some implications of perceived risk', *Employee Relations*, vol. 15, no. 2, pp. 25–32.

AGGLETON, P. and HOMANS, H. (1987) *Educating about AIDS*, Bristol, NHSTA.

AGGLETON, P. (1989) 'Evaluating Health Education about AIDS' in AGGLETON, P., HART, G. and DAVIES, P. (Eds) *AIDS: Social Representations, Social Practices*, London, Falmer Press.

ALEXANDER, P. (1988) 'Prostitutes are being scapegoated for heterosexual AIDS', in DELACOSTE, F. and ALEXANDER, P. (Eds) *Sex Work*, London, Virago.

ALTMAN, D. (1994) *Power and Community: Organizational and Cultural Responses to AIDS*, London, Taylor and Francis.

ANDERMAN, S. (1992) *Labour Law: Management Decisions and Workers' Rights*, London, Butterworth.

ANON (1993) 'Doctors at risk from HIV', anonymous letter to *The Guardian*. 17.4.93.

ARKIN, A. (1994) 'Positive HIV and AIDS policies at work', *Personnel Management*, December, pp. 34–37.

ARMSTRONG, D. (1993) *Political Anatomy of the Body*, Cambridge, Cambridge University Press.

ASHFORTH, B. and HUMPHREY, R. (1993) 'Emotion in the workplace: a reappraisal', paper presented at the British Academy of Management Conference, Milton Keynes, September.

ATKINS, S. and HOGGERT, B. (1984) *Women and the Law*, Oxford, Blackwell.

BAMFORTH, N. (1994) 'Sexual orientation and dismissal', *New Law Journal*, Vol. 14, October.

BANAS, G. (1992) 'Nothing prepared me to manage AIDS', *Harvard Business Review*, July, pp. 26–33.

BARBOUR, R. (1993) 'I Don't Sleep with my Patients — Do You Sleep with Yours?', in AGGLETON, P., DAVIES, P. and HART, G. (Eds) *AIDS: Facing the Second Decade*, London, Falmer.

BARBOUR, R. (1994) 'AIDS Workers and Confidentiality', in AGGLETON, P., DAVIES, P. and HART, G. (Eds) *AIDS: Foundations for the Future*, London, Taylor and Francis.

BELGRAVE, S. (1995) 'One Employer's Approach to Employee Education', in FITZ-SIMONS, D., HARDY, V. and TOLLEY, K. (Eds) *Socio-Economic Impact of AIDS in Europe*, London, Cassell.

BELLOS, A. 'Uganda Determined not to be AIDS Victim' *The Guardian*, 30.11.94.

BENNETT, C. and FERLIE, E. (1994) *Managing Crisis and Change in Health Care*, Buckingham, Open University Press.

BERRIDGE, V. (1992) 'AIDS, the Media and Health Policy', in AGGLETON, P., DAVIES, P. and HART, G. (Eds) *AIDS: Rights, Risk and Reason*, London, Falmer Press.

BLOOR, M. (1995) 'HIV-related Risk Behaviour among International Travellers: An Overview', in FITZSIMONS, D., HARDY, V. and TOLLEY, K. (Eds) *Socio-Economic Impact of AIDS in Europe*, London, Cassell.

BRODIE, D. (1994) *Health Matters at Work*, Eastham, Tudor.

BROWN, H. and SMITH, H. (1992) 'Assertion, not Assimilation: a Feminist Perspective on the Normalization Principle', in BROWN, H. and SMITH, H. (Eds) *Normalization: A Reader for the Nineties*, London, Routledge.

BURRELL, G. (1984) 'Sex and organizational analysis', *Organization Studies*, 5, 2, pp. 97–118.

BURY, J., MORRISON, V. and McLACHLAN, S. (Eds) (1992) *Working with Women and AIDS*, London, Routledge.

BUTCHER, K. (1994) 'Feminists, Prostitutes and HIV', in DOYAL, L., NAIDOO, WILTON, T. (Eds) *AIDS: Setting a Feminist Agenda*, London, Taylor and Francis.

CAMERON, M. (1993) *Living with AIDS*, London, Sage.

CARVEL, J (1992) 'Prison Ends Policy of HIV Segregation', *The Guardian*, 13.1.92.

CLARK, D. (ed) *The Sociology of Death*, Oxford, Blackwell.

COCKBURN, C. (1989) 'Equal opportunities: the short and long agenda', *Industrial Relations Journal*, 44, pp. 213–225.

COCKBURN, C. (1991) *In the Way of Women*, Basingstoke, Macmillan.

COCKCROFT, A. (1991) 'Testing patients for HIV antibodies is useful for infection control purposes', *Reviews in Medical Virology*, 1, pp. 5–9.

COLLINSON, D. (1991) 'Poachers turned gamekeepers: are personnel managers one of the barriers to equal opportunities?', *Human Resource Management Journal*, 1, 3, pp. 58–76.

COLLINSON, D. (1992) *Managing the Shopfloor*, Berlin, Walter de Gruyter.

COLLINSON, D., KNIGHTS, D. and COLLINSON, M. (1990) *Managing to Discriminate*, London, Routledge.

COTTON, T. and KUMARI, V. (1990) 'Local Authorities and HIV-related Illness', in AGGLETON, P., DAVIES, P. and HART, G. (Eds) *AIDS: Individual, Cultural and Policy Dimensions*, London, Falmer Press.

DALE, A. (1987) 'Occupational inequality, gender and life-cycle', *Work Employment and Society*, 1, 3, pp. 326–351.

DAVIES, P. and SIMPSON, P. (1990) 'On male homosexual prostitution and HIV', in AGGLETON, P., DAVIES, P. and HART, G. (Eds) *AIDS: Individual, Cultural and Policy Dimensions*, London, Falmer Press.

DIAMANT, L. (Ed.) (1993) *Homosexual Issues in the Workplace*, London, Taylor and Francis, pp. 243–264.

DOCKRELL, M. (1994) 'AIDS and The Enemy', *The Guardian*, 3.12.94.

DODD, V. and NELSON, D. (1994) 'Harrods Workers' Fury over Illegal HIV Tests', *The Observer*, 17.4.94.

DOE/HSE (1987) *AIDS and the Workplace*, London, Department of Employment/ Health and Safety Executive.

DORA (1993) *Digest of Organizational Responses to AIDS*, **2**, 3, May, p. 12.

DOUGLAS, M. (1991) *Purity and Danger*, London, Routledge.

ELFORD, J. and COCKCROFT, A. (1991) 'Compulsory HIV antibody testing, universal precautions and the perceived risk of HIV' *AIDS Care*, **3**, 2, pp. 151–58.

EMERSON, E. (1992) 'What is Normalization?', in BROWN, H. and SMITH, H. (Eds) *Normalization: A Reader for the Nineties*, London, Routledge.

EOC (1987) *Formal Investigation Report: Dan AIR*, London, Equal Opportunities Commission, January.

EU (1991) 'European Commission Recommendation on the protection of the dignity of men and women at work' and 'Code of practice on measures to combat sexual harassment', in *Official Journal of the European Communities*, Brussels, L 49/ 1–49/7.

EUROPEAN COMMISSION (1990) *Resolution of the Council and Ministers for Health of the Member States on the Fight Against AIDS*, Social Europe, January.

FELDMAN, S. (1991) 'The AIDS epidemic: three successful programmes', *Personnel*, **68**, 4.

FERNS, P. (1992) 'Promoting Race Equality through Normalization', in BROWN, H. and SMITH, H. (Eds) *Normalization: A Reader for the Nineties*, London, Routledge.

FINEMAN, S. (Ed.) (1993) *Emotion in Organizations*, London, Sage.

FITZPATRICK, P. (1987) 'Racism and the innocence of law', *Journal of Legal Studies*, **14**, 1, pp. 119–132.

FOX, A. (1974) *Beyond Contract*, Oxford, Blackwell.

FRANCIS, J. (1993) 'Erosion process', *Community Care*, March, pp. 16–17.

GAYMER, J. (1989) 'The Legal Position', in 'HIV/AIDS in Employment', unpublished booklet, National AIDS Trust, London.

GINN, J. and ARBER, S. (1993) 'Pension penalties: the gendered division of occupational welfare', *Work Employment and Society*, **7**, 1, pp. 47–70.

GOFFMAN, E. (1963) *Stigma*, London, Prentice Hall.

GONSIOREK, J. (1993) 'Threat, Stress and Adjustment: Mental Health and the Workplace for Gay and Lesbian Individuals', in DIAMANT, L. (Ed.) *Homosexual Issues in the Workplace*, London, Taylor and Francis.

GOSS, D. (1993) 'The ethics of HIV/AIDS in the workplace', *Business Ethics: A European Review*, **2**, 3, pp. 143–148.

GOSS, D. (1994a) 'Writing about AIDS: framing policy', paper presented at the EIASM Workshop on Writing, Rationality and Organization, Brussels, April.

GOSS, D. (1994b) 'Health at work: HRM and greedy institutions', paper presented at the Strategic Directions in HRM Conference, Nottingham Trent University, December.

GREEN, G. (1995) 'Processes of Stigmatization and Impact on Employment of People with HIV', in FITZSIMONS, D., HARDY, V. and TOLLEY, K. (Eds) *Socio-Economic Impact of AIDS in Europe*, London, Cassell.

GREENSLADE, M. (1991) 'Managing diversity: lessons from the United States', *Personnel Management*, December.

GREGORY, J. and O'DONOVAN, K. (1985) *Sexual Divisions in Law*, London, Weidenfeld and Nicolson.

GREGORY, J. (1987) *Sex, Race and the Law: Legislating for Equality*, London, Sage.

GUTEK, B. (1989) 'Sexuality in the workplace: key issues in social research and organization practice' in HEARN, J., SHEPPARD, D., TANCRED-SHERIFF, P. and BURRELL, G. (Eds), *The Sexuality of Organization*, London, Sage.

HAKIM, C. (1992) 'Grateful slaves and self-made women', *European Sociological Review*, **2**, 2, pp. 157–188.

HAKIM, C. (1994) 'The myth of rising female employment', *Work Employment and Society*, **7**, 1, pp. 97–120.

HALFORD, S. (1992) 'Feminist Change in a Patriarchal Organization', in SAVAGE, M. and WITZ, A. (Eds) *Gender and Bureaucracy*, Oxford, Blackwell.

HAMILTON, J. (1987) 'The AIDS epidemic and business', *Business Week*, March, pp. 122–24.

HARRIS, D. (1990) 'AIDS and employment' in HARRIS, D. and HAIGH, R. (Eds) *AIDS: A Guide to the Law*, London, Routledge.

HEARN, J. and PARKIN, W. (1987) *Sex at Work: The Power and Paradox of Organization Sexuality*, Brighton, Wheatsheaf.

HEARN, J. and PARKIN, W. (1994) 'Sexuality, gender and organizations: acknowledging complexities and contentions', paper presented at the British Sociological Association Conference, University of Central Lancashire, April.

HEPPLE, B. (1979) *Hepple and O'Higgins Employment Law*, London, Sweet and Maxwell, 3rd edition.

HEREK, G. and GLUNT, E. (1991) 'AIDS-related attitudes in the US', *Journal of Sex Research*, **28**, 1, pp. 91–123.

HICKSON, F., WEATHERBURN, P., HOWS, J. and DAVIES, P. (1994) 'Selling Safer Sex: Male Masseurs and Escorts in the UK', in AGGLETON, P., DAVIES, P. and HART, G. (Eds) *AIDS: Foundations for the Future*, London, Taylor and Francis.

HOLMYARD, E. (1993) 'From Prejudice to Policy: HIV/AIDS Issues and Employment', unpublished MSc dissertation, University of Southampton.

HSW (1990) 'AIDS and the workplace', *Health and Safety at Work*, p. 15, January.

HUSSEY, J. (1995) 'HIV and AIDS: a personal consideration of the principle of employer interest', in FITZSIMONS, D., HARDY, V. and TOLLEY, K. (Eds) *Socio-Economic Impact of AIDS in Europe*, London, Cassell.

IDS (1987) *AIDS and Employment*, Incomes Data Services Study 393, September.

IDS (1993a) *AIDS Returns to the Agenda*, Incomes Data Services Study 528, April.

IDS (1993b) *Sex Discrimination*, Incomes Data Services Employment Law Handbook, Series 2, London, IDS.

IRS (1991) 'AIDS at the workplace 1/2' *Health and Safety Information Bulletin 187/7*, Industrial Relations Service.

JACKSON, H. and PITTS, M. (1991) 'Company policy on AIDS in Zimbabwe', *Journal of Social development in Africa*, **6**, 2, pp. 53–70.

JAMES, N. (1993) 'Divisions of emotional labour: disclosure and cancer' in FINEMAN, S. (Ed.) *Emotion in Organizations*, London, Sage.

JOHNSTONE, V. (1992) 'How should we respond to AIDS?', *Sunday Telegraph*, 29.3.92.

JURY, L. (1993) 'Gays suffering high level of harassment', *The Guardian*, 20.11.93.

KANDOLA, R. and FULLERTON, J. (1994a) 'Diversity: more than an empty slogan', *Personnel Management*, November, pp. 46–50.

KANDOLA, R. and FULLERTON, J. (1994b) *Managing the Mosaic*, London, IPM.

KEAY, D. and LEACH, M. (1993) 'Positive thinking about HIV', *Human Resources*, Spring, pp. 36–40.

KELLY, J. (1989) 'The AIDS virus in the workplace', *The Transnational Lawyer*, **12**, 2.

KELLY, J. (1992) 'HIV and AIDS and the workplace', *Labour Law Journal*, December, pp. 759–73.

KINNEL, H. (1991) 'Prostitutes' perceptions of risk and factors related to risk-taking', in AGGLETON, P., HART, G. and DAVIES, P. (Eds) *AIDS: Responses, Interventions and Care*, London, Falmer Press.

KIRP, D. (1989) 'Uncommon decency: Pacific Bell responds to AIDS', *Harvard Business Review*, May, pp. 140–51.

KNIGHTS, D. and MORGAN, G. (1990) 'The concept of strategy in sociology: a note of dissent', *Sociology*, **24**, 3, pp. 475–484.

KOHL, J., MILLER, A. and BARTON, L. (1990) 'Levi's corporate AIDS programme', *Long Range Planning*, **23**, 6, pp. 31–34.

KOLB, D. and PUTNAM, J. (Eds) (1992) *Hidden Conflict in Organizations*, London, Sage.

LAGER (1990) *HIV and AIDS: Guidelines for Voluntary Organizations and Small Employers*, London, Lesbian and Gay Employment Rights.

LAGER (1992) *HIV and AIDS: Continued Employment Guidelines for Employers*, London, Lesbian and Gay Employment Rights.

LEE, J. and BROWN, R. (1993) 'Hiring, firing and promoting', in DIAMANT, L. (Ed.) *Homosexual Issues in the Workplace*, London, Taylor and Francis.

LEGGE, K. (1989) 'HRM: a critical analysis', in STOREY, J. (Ed.) *New Developments in HRM*, London, Routledge.

LESSLIE, T. (1994) 'HIV list passed to health authority', *The Pink Paper*, 11.2.94.

LEWIS, P. (1981) 'An analysis of why legislation has failed to provide employment protection for unfairly dismissed employees', *British Journal of Industrial Relations*, **29**, 3, pp. 361–23.

LIPPMAN, H. (1992) 'HIV and professional ethics: nurses speak out', *Registered Nurse*, June, pp. 28–32.

LONSDALE, S. (1990) *Women and Disability*, Basingstoke, Macmillan.

LUPTON, D. (1994a) *Moral Threats and Dangerous Desires: AIDS in the News Media*, London, Taylor and Francis.

LUPTON, D. (1994b) *Medicine as Culture*, London, Sage.

MACIVER, N. (1992) 'Developing a Service for Prostitutes in Glasgow', in BURY, J., MORRISON, V. and MCLACHLAN, S.(Eds) *Working with Women and AIDS*, London, Routledge.

MACLAGAN, P. and SNELL, R. (1992) 'Some implications for management development of research into manager's moral dilemmas', *British Journal of Management*, **3**, 3, pp. 157–68.

MARQUET, J., HUBERT, M. and CAMPENHOUDT, L. (1995) 'Public Awareness of AIDS: Discrimination and the Effects of Mistrust', in FITZSIMONS, D., HARDY, V. and TOLLEY, K. (Eds) *Socio-Economic Impact of AIDS in Europe*, London, Cassell.

MELLOR, P. and SCHILLING, C. (1993) 'Modernity, self-identity and the sequestration of death', *Sociology*, **27**, 3, pp. 411–32.

MERSON, M. (1995) 'AIDS: epidemic update and corporate responses' in FITZSIMONS, D., HARDY, V. and TOLLEY, K. (Eds) *Socio-Economic Impact of AIDS in Europe*, London, Cassell.

MILLS, A. and MURGATROYD, S. (1991) *Organizational Rules*, Buckingham, OUP.

MORGAN THOMAS, R. (1990) 'AIDS Risk, Alcohol, Drugs and the Sex Industry', in PLANT, M. (Ed.) *AIDS, Drugs and Prostitution*, London, Routledge.

MORGAN THOMAS, R. (1992) 'HIV and the Sex Industry' in BURY, J., MORRISON, V. and McLACHLAN, S. (Eds) *Working With Women and AIDS*, London, Routledge, pp. 71–84.

MORRIS, J. (1993) *Pride Against Prejudice*, London, The Women's Press.

MULHOLLAND, M. (1993) 'AIDS, HIV and the health care worker', *Professional Negligence*, **9**, 2, pp. 79–84.

NATIONAL AIDS TRUST (1992) *Companies Act!*, London, National AIDS Trust.

NIRJE, B. (1980) 'The Normalization Principle', in FLYNN, R. and NITSCH, K. (Eds) *Normalization, Social Integration and Community Services*, Baltimore, University Park Press.

PANOS (1990) *The Third Epidemic: Repercussions of the fear of AIDS*, London, Panos Publications.

PATTON, C. (1990) *Inventing AIDS*, London, Routledge.

PATTON, C. (1994) *Last Served? Gendering the HIV Pandemic*, London, Taylor and Francis.

Personnel Management Plus (1994) 'Occupational nurses pressured to disclose confidential records' *Personnel Management Plus*, September, p. 1.

PETTIGREW, A., FERLIE, E., and McKEE, L. (1992) *Shaping Strategic Change: Making Change in Large Organizations — the Case of the NHS*, London, Sage.

PIERRET, J. (1992) 'Coping with AIDS in everyday life', in POLLAK, M., PAICHELER, G. and PIERRET, J. (Eds) *AIDS: A Problem for Sociological Research*, London, Sage.

PLANT, M. (1990) 'Sex work, alcohol, drugs and AIDS', in PLANT, M. (Ed.) *AIDS, Drugs and Prostitution*, London, Routledge.

PLANT, M. and PLANT, M. (1992) *Risk-Takers*, London, Routledge.

RICHARDSON, D. (1994) 'Inclusions and Exclusions: Lesbians, HIV and AIDS', in DOYAL, L., NAIDOO, J. and WILTON, T. (Eds) *AIDS: Setting a Feminist Agenda*, London, Taylor and Francis.

RIEBEN SCHIZAS, A. (1995) 'Employment, the Law and HIV: An Overview of European Legislation', in FITZSIMONS, D., HARDY, V. and TOLLEY, K. (Eds) *Socio-Economic Impact of AIDS in Europe*, London, Cassell.

ROBERTSON, H. (1987) 'AIDS — a Trade Union Issue', in AGGLETON, P. and HOMANS, H. (Eds) *Social Aspects of AIDS*, London, Falmer Press.

ROBINSON, T. and DAVIES, P. (1991) 'London's Homosexual Male Prostitutes: Power, Peer Groups and HIV', in AGGLETON, P., HART, G. and DAVIES, P. (Eds) *AIDS: Responses, Interventions and Care*, London, Falmer Press.

ROSS, M. (1993) 'Mental Health Issues and the Worker with AIDS' in DIAMANT, L. (Ed.) *Homosexual Issues in the Workplace*, London, Taylor and Francis.

SCAMBLER, G. and GRAHAM-SMITH, R. (1992) 'Female Prostitution and AIDS: The Realities of Social Exclusion', in AGGLETON, P., DAVIES, P. and HART, G. (Eds) *AIDS: Rights, Risk and Reason*, London, Falmer Press.

SCHRAMM-EVANS, Z. (1990) 'Responses to AIDS, 1986–1987', in AGGLETON, P., DAVIES, P. and HART, G. (Eds) *AIDS: Individual, Cultural and Policy Dimensions*, London, Falmer Press.

SHANSON, D. and COCKCROFT, A. (1991) 'Testing patients for antibodies is useful for infection control purposes', *Reviews in Medical Virology*, 1, pp. 5–9.

SHAW, M. (1990) 'Strategy and social process: military context and sociological analysis', *Sociology*, **24**, 3, pp. 465–74.

SHEARER, A. (1981) *Disability: Whose Handicap?*, Oxford, Blackwell.

SIEVERS, B. (1993) 'Love in the time of AIDS', paper presented at the 11 International SCOS Conference, Barcelona.

SIM, J. (1992) 'AIDS, nursing and occupational risk: an ethical analysis', *Journal of Advanced Nursing*, 17, pp. 569–575.

SMALL, N. (1993) 'Dying in a Public Space: AIDS Deaths', in CLARK, D. (Ed.) *The Sociology of Death*, Oxford, Blackwell.

SMITHURST, M. (1990) 'AIDS: risks and discrimination', in ALMOND, B. (Ed.) *AIDS A Moral Issue*, Basingstoke, Macmillan.

SOM (1992) *What Employers Should Know About HIV and AIDS*, London, Society of Occupational Medicine.

SONTAG, S. (1991) *Illness and Metaphor. AIDS and its Metaphors*, London, Penguin.

SOUTHAM, C. and HOWARD, G. (1988) *AIDS and Employment Law*, London, Financial Training Publications.

SULLIVAN, S. (1991) 'The AIDS epidemic: how the insurance industry has responded', *Life Association News*, February, pp. 59–62.

SWISS INSTITUTE OF COMPARATIVE LAW (1993) *Discrimination Against Persons with HIV or AIDS*, Strasbourg, Council of Europe.

TGWU (undated) *Information and Advice about AIDS*, London, TGWU.

TOFFLER, B. (1986) *Tough Choices: Managers Talk Ethics*, New York, J Wiley.

VEKSNER, L. and LANE, A. (1993) 'Bud Medicine', *The Guardian*, 17.4.93.

VEST, J., O'BRIEN, F. and VEST, M. (1991) 'AIDS training in the workplace', *Training and Development*, December, pp. 59–64.

WALSH, G. (1992) 'AIDS: fear of contagion among nurses', *British Journal of Nursing*, 1, 2, p. 67.

WATNEY, S. (1987) 'AIDS, Moral Panic Theory and Homophobia', in AGGLETON, P. and HOMAN, H. (Eds) *Social Aspects of AIDS*, London, Falmer Press.

WATNEY, S. (1989) 'The Subject of AIDS', in AGGLETON, P., HART, G. and DAVIES, P. (Eds) *AIDS: Social Representations, Social Practices*, London, Falmer Press.

WATT, R. (1992) 'HIV. Discrimination, unfair dismissal and pressure to dismiss', *Industrial Law Journal*, **21**, 4, pp. 280–92.

WEEKS, J. (1991) *Against Nature*, London, River Oram.

WESTERHALL, L. and SALDEEN, A. (1992) 'Some reflections on HIV/AIDS law in Sweden', in *Law and AIDS: an International Comparison*, Paris, CNRS.

WILSON, P. (1992) *HIV and AIDS in the Workplace*, London, National AIDS Trust.

WILSON, P. (1993) 'The Transformation of HIV-related Problems in the Voluntary Sector', in AGGLETON, P., DAVIES, P. and HART, G. (Eds) *AIDS: Facing the Second Decade*, London, Falmer Press.

WILSON, P. (1994) 'Colleague or viral vector? The legal construction of the HIV positive worker', *Law and Policy*, Fall issue.

WILSON, P. (1995) 'Discrimination in the Workplace: Protection and the Law in the UK', in FITZSIMONS, D., HARDY, V. and TOLLEY, K. (Eds) *Socio-Economic Impact of AIDS in Europe*, London, Cassell.

WILTON, T. (1992) *Antibody Politic*, Cheltenham, Clarion.

WOLFENSBERGER, W. (1972) *The Principle of Normalization in Human Services*, Toronto, NIMR.

WOLFENSBERGER, W. (1983) 'Social role valorization', *Mental Retardation*, 34, pp. 22–25.

WOLFENSBERGER, W. and THOMAS, S. (1983) *PASSING: Program Analysis of Service Systems Implementation of Normalization Goals*, Toronto, NIMR.

WOLFENSBERGER, W. and TULLMAN, S. (1989) 'A Brief Outline of the Principle of Normalization', in BRECHIN, A. and WALMSLEY, J. (Eds) *Making Connections*, Milton Keynes, Open University Press.

Index